Flexible
Fitness Guide

Disclosure Agreements

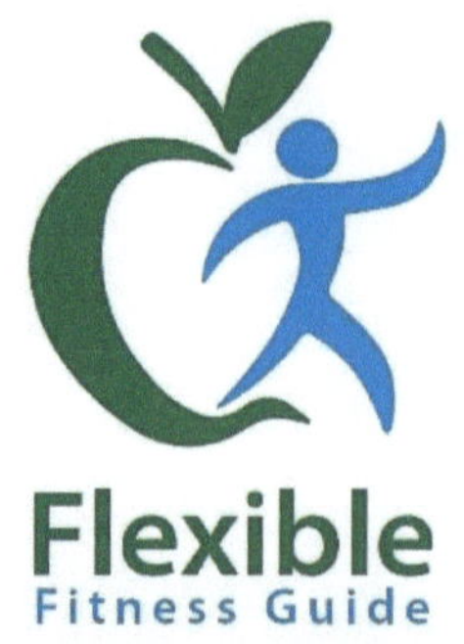

By purchasing and/or receiving this fitness and nutrition book from Daniel Shpigel, hereafter referred to as "SELLER," you, as the purchaser and/or receiver of this book, hereafter referred to as "BUYER," automatically agree to the following conditions:

I. NO DISTRIBUTION OR RESALE RIGHTS

BUYER understands that this book is copyrighted and that any distribution, including without limitation, resale of this book, whether for profit or non-profit, is strictly prohibited. BUYER understands that any distribution or resale of this book, in any form, is a violation of the SELLER'S intellectual property rights that will cause irreparable and continuing damage to SELLER for which money damages are insufficient, and SELLER shall be entitled to injunctive relief and/or a decree for specific performance, and such other relief as may be proper (including money damages).

In addition to the SELLER being able to seek money damages from the Arbitrator or Court for any such breach of disclosure, BUYER also agrees to automatically pay SELLER a sum of $100,000.00 (USD) by default. Both parties agree that SELLER's book could have a high marketable value and that $100,000.00 is a reasonable amount to partially help make SELLER whole again for any such breach.

II. MEDICAL DISCLAIMER

BUYER acknowledges that this book does not provide medical advice, diagnosis, or treatment, nor is the SELLER necessarily a health professional.

The contents of this book are for informational purposes only. The content is not intended to be a substitute for professional medical advice, diagnosis, or treatment.

Always seek the advice of your physician or other qualified health providers with any questions you may have regarding a medical condition. Never disregard professional medical advice or delay in seeking it because of something you have read in this book. If you think you may have a medical emergency, call your doctor or emergency services immediately.

Reliance on any information provided by this book is solely at your own risk.

III. INDEMNIFCATION

I, the BUYER, hereby understand and acknowledge that the content regarding fitness and nutrition in this book may expose me to inherent risks, including accidents, injuries (mental and physical), illness, or even death. I, BUYER, assume all risk of injuries associated with such participation, including, but not limited to, falls, physical injuries, mental trauma and psychological injuries, and all other such risks, whether known or unknown.

In consideration of the purchase and/or receipt of this book., I, BUYER, agree, for myself and anyone entitled to act on my behalf, to **HOLD HARMLESS, WAIVE, INDEMNIFY, AND RELEASE** SELLER or any of SELLER's officers, agents, employees, organizers, representatives, and successors from any responsibility, liabilities, demands, or claims of any kind arising out of any injury, illness, or lack of results that arise from reading and following the instructions in this book.

IV. COPYRIGHT NOTICE

Copyright © 2018 by Daniel Shpigel

All rights reserved. No part of this publication may be reproduced, distributed, or transmitted in any form or by any means, including photocopying, recording, or other electronic or mechanical methods, without the prior written permission of the author, except in the case of brief quotations embodied in critical reviews and certain other noncommercial uses permitted by copyright law. For permission requests, write to the publisher, addressed "Attention: Daniel Shpigel" at the email address dshpig@gmail.com.

V. JURISDICTION AND ATTORNEY FEES

By purchasing or receiving this book, BUYER irrevocably agrees that this disclosure shall be governed in all respects by the laws governed by and construed in accordance with the laws of the County of Philadelphia and the State of Pennsylvania, even if the BUYER is outside that jurisdiction. If a proceeding is commenced to resolve any dispute that arises between the parties with respect to the matters covered by this disclosure, the prevailing party in such proceeding shall be entitled to receive its reasonable attorneys' fees, expert witness fees and out of pocket costs incurred in connection with such proceeding, in addition to any other relief to which such prevailing party may be entitled.

Table of Contents

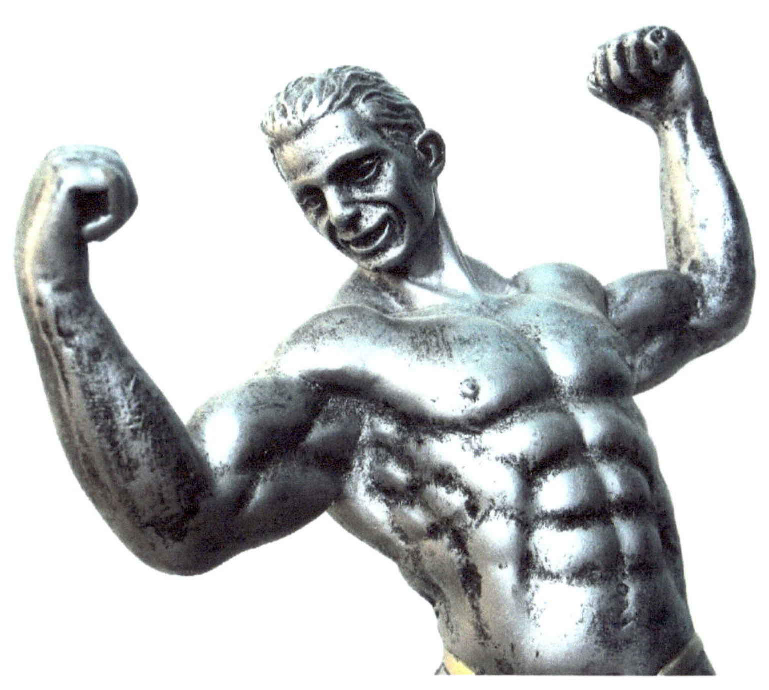

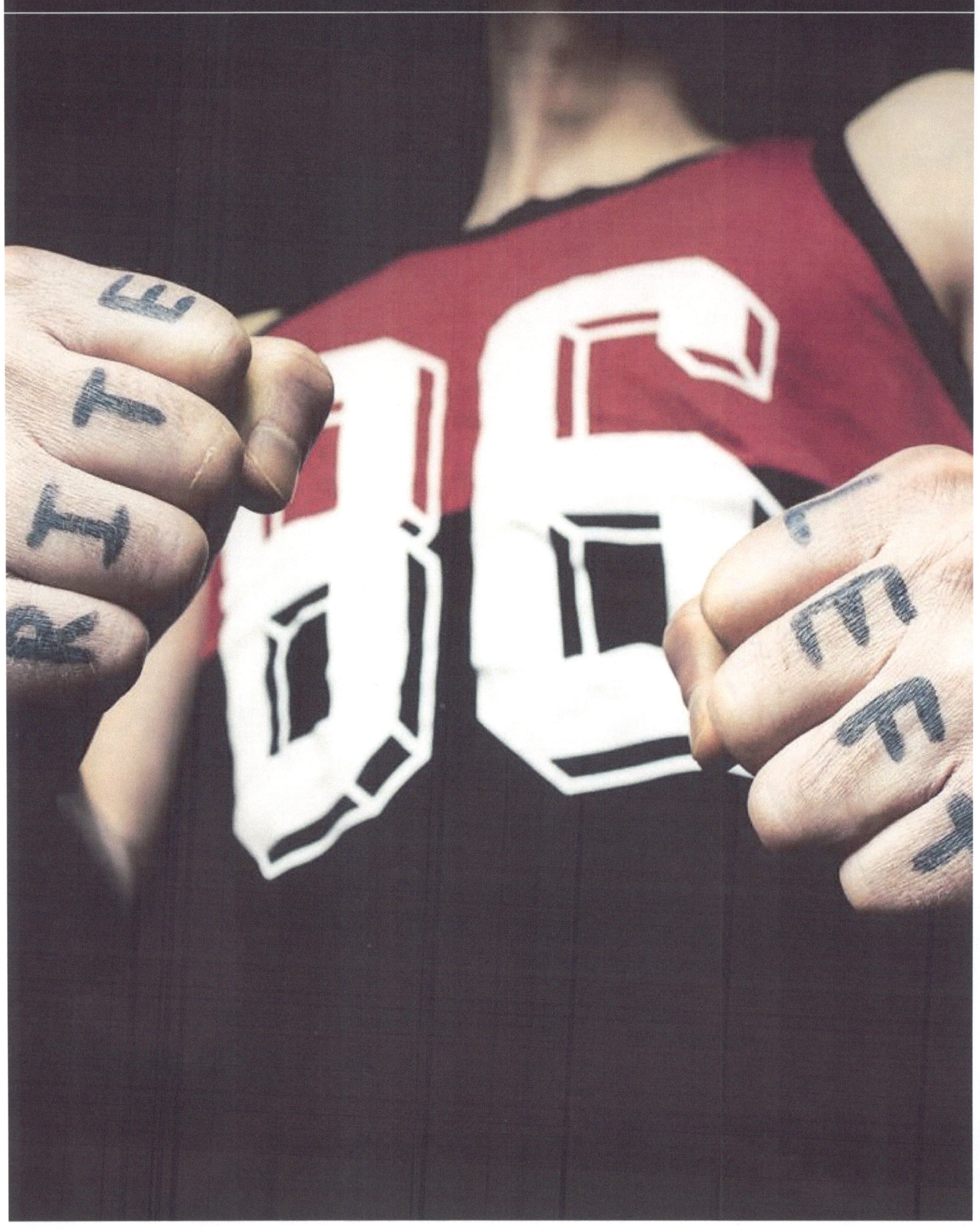

Daniel Shpigel
Author, Editor and Designer

Bodybuilding and nutrition have been passions of mine since I was a teenager; to date, my passion has not faded even a little. The information that Nabel and I convey in this book is the culmination of knowledge gained through our practice of nutrition and well-being. It is important to embrace the lifestyle of fitness and to allow your mind, body and soul to adapt accordingly.

I am currently enrolled as a medical student and hope to apply my education to bodybuilding in order to bust myths and highlight what truly can help you achieve your goals. A big issue we face in healthcare today is chronic illness that is treated and not cured; many of these illnesses are greatly improved by lifestyle modifications such as diet and exercise. This book equips readers with the knowledge to comfortably set physique goals, calculate nutritional requirements and establish a personal diet plan.

While I am crunched for time, I still find the motivation to stick to both our workout and nutritional guidelines. Remember, I advocate *flexible* fitness. Success is a journey, not a destination!

Nabel Khatut
Author and Motivator

I was first introduced to bodybuilding during my teenage years in Dubai; I worshipped pioneers like Arnold Schwarzenegger and Aziz "Zyzz" Shavershian. During my undergraduate studies, I became serious about my own strength and physique, and my craving for the sport of bodybuilding truly took effect.

After years of independent study I decided to pursue a Master's degree in nutrition and I am currently enrolled in a prestigious university. I truly love nutrition because I believe in the cliché phrase, "you are what you eat." Truly, by manipulating our diet and putting our bodies under calculated stress, we have the ability to look and feel however we want.

With the information we've gathered, I'm able to manipulate my weight, muscle and fat mass, and physique month to month with relatively few deviation from my plans. My goal is to convey as much useful knowledge and as little extraneous information as possible in our writing. Now go out there, put this guide and your body to the test, and get what you deserve!

Why Flexible Fitness?

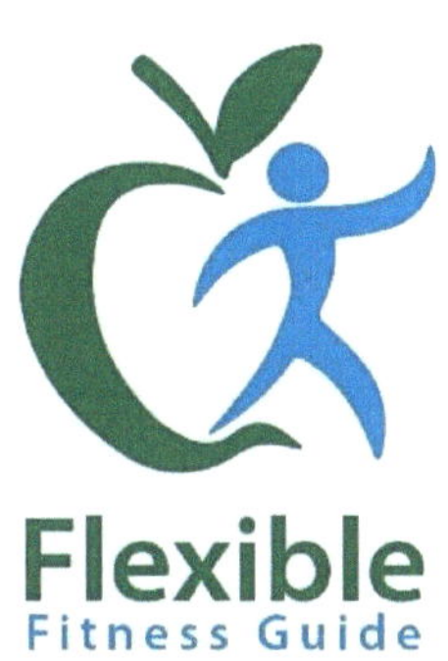

Flexible
Fitness Guide

This is the Internet Age; everyone is set on the instantaneous – from immediate answers on Google to immediate sharing on social media and instant gratification via bells and whistles when you advance a level on Bejeweled. We're here to tell you to forget about instant gratification when it comes to physical fitness.

We believe in the type of physical fitness and well-being that is goal oriented and lasts a lifetime. This certainly does not mean sacrificing your favorite food or spending half of your day exercising. Our approaches will give you the tools you need to achieve your goals whether that is putting on tons of muscle mass or shredding a few pounds to fit into your old wedding dress.

Through exposure to people inside and out of the fitness world, it became apparent to us that many people aspire to become physically fit but simply do not know where to start. The bulk of information on the internet is frankly confusing. Often times it is hard to tell whether it is fact, opinion or just a complete gimmick. Some of you might want to have six-pack abs while others simply want to lose a few pounds and feel healthier. Some of you are hard-gainers and want to add quality pounds of muscle to your frame while others are struggling to lose that holiday weight. We will give you the quality information you need to set realistic goals and cater the program you need to achieve them.

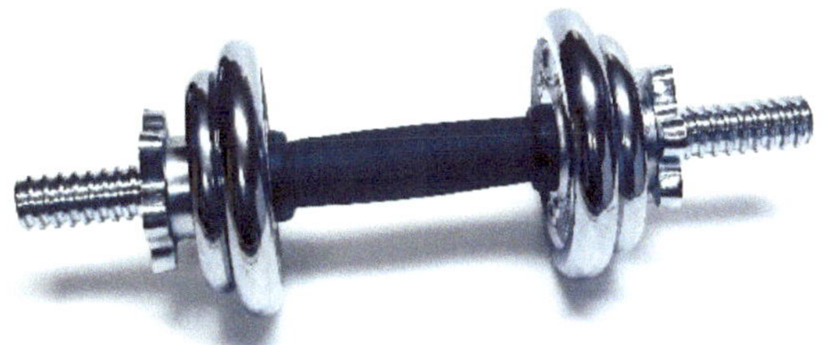

Why Flexible Fitness?

Our mission is to help you acquire the physique that you desire by providing you with comprehensive yet easy to understand guides on workout and nutrition. No matter what your desired physique is, you'll be able to take a stride in the right direction by following our programs.

Remember, we don't believe in short-term gimmicks that "turn your life around in 30 days." We believe in a lifestyle of **flexible fitness**. You have to be willing to embrace a lifestyle of fitness. This does not have to happen overnight, but the greater commitment you make to a healthy lifestyle the easier it will be to achieve and maintain your goals.

Inflexible programs that ask you to eat an unrealistic number of calories or exercise for an inordinate amount of time every day are unsustainable. We believe in flexibility and enjoyment of life as part of leading a fit and healthy lifestyle. Do not skip out on dinner with friends because your diet doesn't allow it. Do not skip out on a weekend getaway because you are worried that you cannot get to the gym in that time frame. Go out to dinner and choose your food so that it fits your macronutrient count. Go on that getaway and either find a way to get in your exercise or make up for it at a more convenient time. Being flexible is what will allow you to embrace the lifestyle and enjoy your journey to physical fitness.

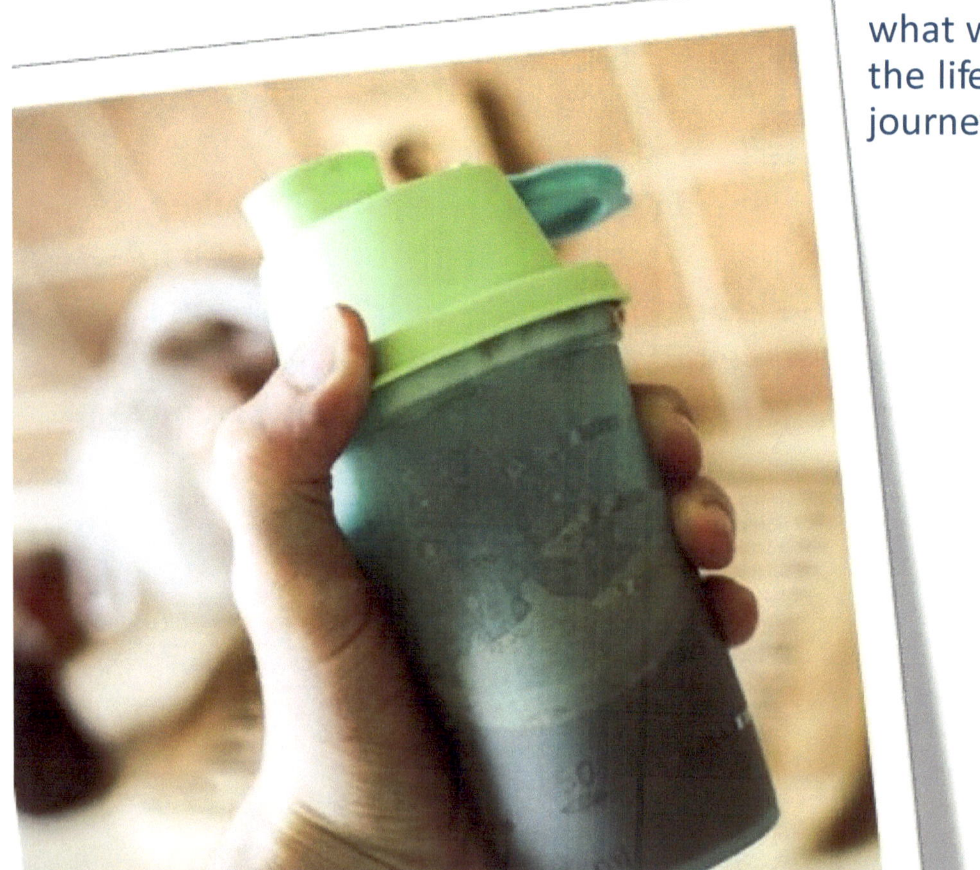

What Results Can I Expect?

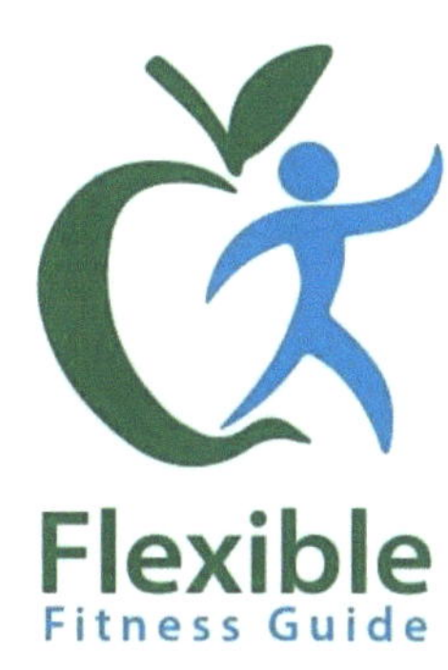

The answer to this question depends on you. If you dedicate yourself to following this program and make a conscious effort to perfect your workout routine, you will come closer to achieving your goals! You will face challenges and might get frustrated at times. You need to stay focused and keep a positive mentality. Setting an attainable goal for yourself and knowing exactly how you plan to achieve it will help you stay motivated; those plans are exactly what we hope to provide you with.

Chapter 1
Calculating BMR and TDEE

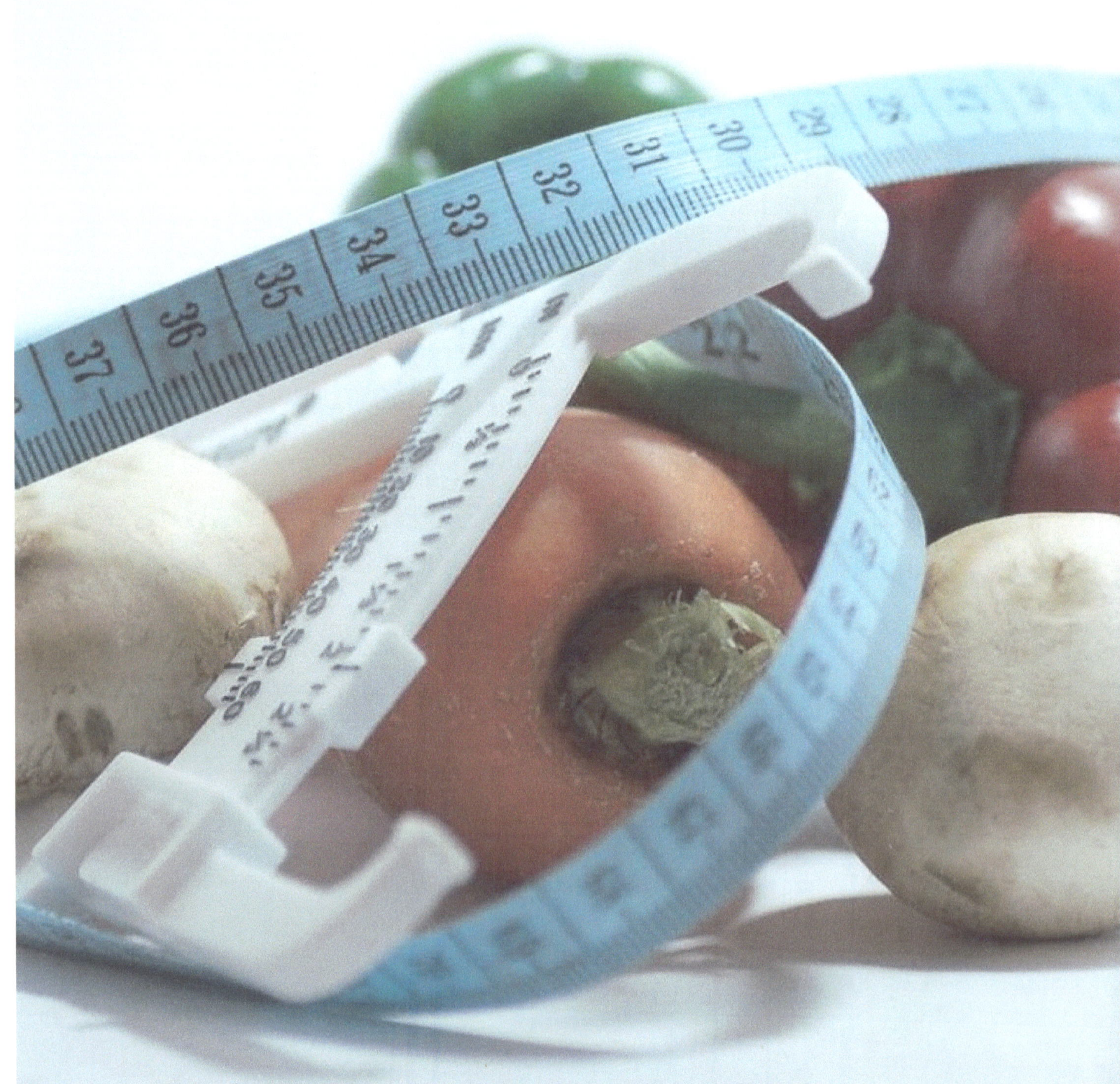

Basal Metabolic Rate

The first step to crafting your own personal meal plan is to calculate your **basal metabolic rate**, or BMR. <u>Your BMR is the number of kilocalories (simply referred to as "calories," colloquially) that your body uses daily to perform essential functions</u>; this, of course, excludes the physical activity that you perform, for instance, in the gym — but we'll get there. You might be thinking to yourself, "I did not sign up for an algebra class; just tell me how to manipulate my weight the way I want to!" In order to come up with a nutrition plan that will allow you to manipulate your weight the way you want, you *must* know the energy that you use on a daily basis.

Weight gain and loss boils down to the calories you take in versus the calories you burn.

The next few chapters will clarify exactly why these measurements are necessary, and it will explain the importance of a concept that should really stick with you long after you read this book:

CALORIES IN

VERSUS

CALORIES OUT

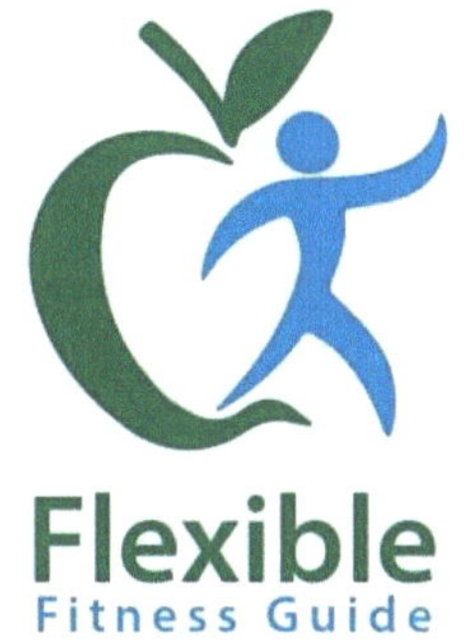

Flexible
Fitness Guide

Basal Metabolic Rate

Let's get started with your BMR. Firstly, if you follow the imperial system and measure your weight in pounds and your height in inches, you need to convert those figures to kilograms and centimeters, respectively.

Conversion from Pounds to Kilograms

$$\text{weight in kilograms} = \frac{\text{weight in pounds}}{2.2}$$

Conversion from Inches to Centimeters

$$\text{height in centimeters} = \text{height in inches} \times 2.54$$

For the sake of providing an example, we will use Arnold Columbu as our subject. Arnold weighs 190 pounds and is 5 feet 9 inches (69 inches) tall. We need to convert these figures to kilograms and centimeters.

Conversion from Pounds to Kilograms

$$86.4 \text{ kilograms} = \frac{190 \text{ pounds}}{2.2}$$

Conversion from Inches to Centimeters

$$175.3 \text{ centimeters} = 69 \text{ inches} \times 2.54$$

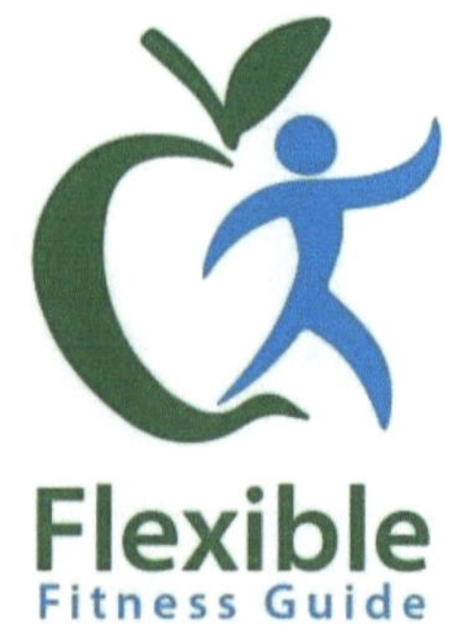

Basal Metabolic Rate

The formulas for calculating BMR are slightly different for men and women. To be clear, perform the calculations contained inside the parentheses first, then add or subtract the products of those calculations. Try using our example below for practice.

BMR for Men (kg, cm)

$$BMR = 88.3 + (13.4 \times \text{weight}) + (4.8 \times \text{height}) - (5.7 \times \text{age})$$

BMR for Women (kg, cm)

$$BMR = 447.6 + (9.2 \times \text{weight}) + (3.1 \times \text{height}) - (4.3 \times \text{age})$$

We will continue using Arnold's measurements to calculate his BMR, as an example. Arnold is 22 years of age. He weighs 86.4 kg and is 175.3 centimeters tall.

Arnold's BMR

$$88.3 + (13.4 \text{x} 86.4 \text{kg}) + (4.8 \text{x} 175.3 \text{cm}) - (5.7 \text{x} 22) = 1{,}962 \text{ calories}$$

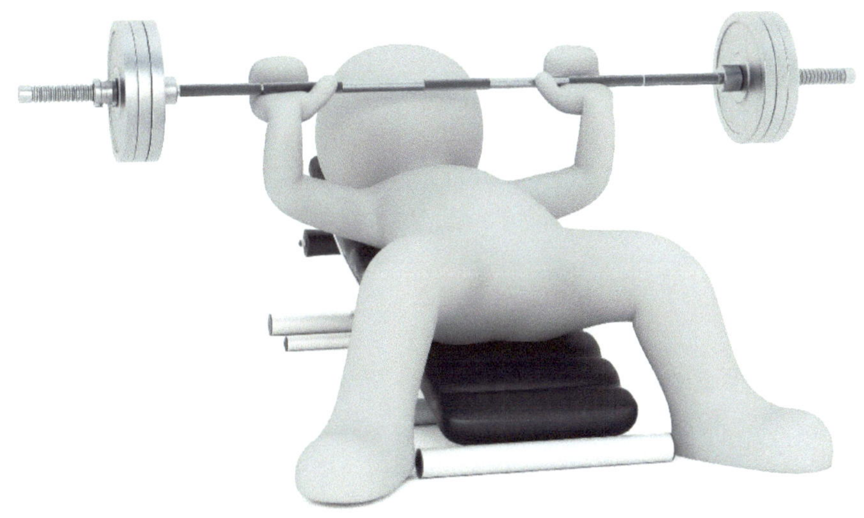

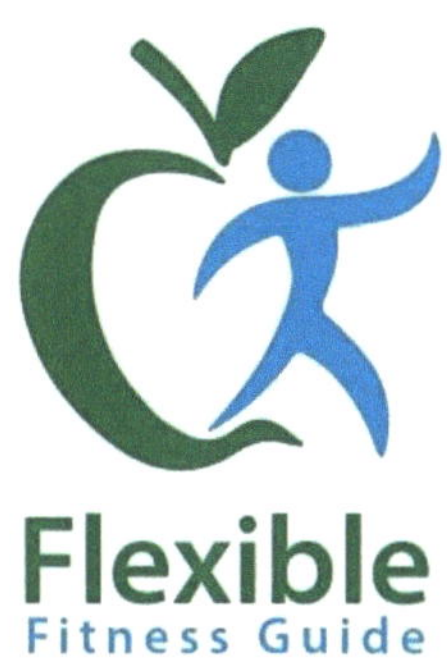

Total Daily Energy Expenditure

The second step is to calculate your **total daily energy expenditure**, or TDEE. <u>This is your BMR adjusted for daily activities</u>. This is where we take into account your activity level, including the number of times you exercise per week, the type of job you work, etc. The table on this page will help you determine the multiplier that you should use for the calculations on the following page.

Activity Level	Activity Factor
Sedentary: light or no exercise and desk job	1.2
Lightly Active: light exercise or sports 1-3 days a week	1.375
Moderately Active: moderate exercise or sports 3-5 days a week	1.55
Very Active: hard exercise or sports 6-7 days a week	1.725
Extremely Active: hard daily exercise or sports and physical job	1.9

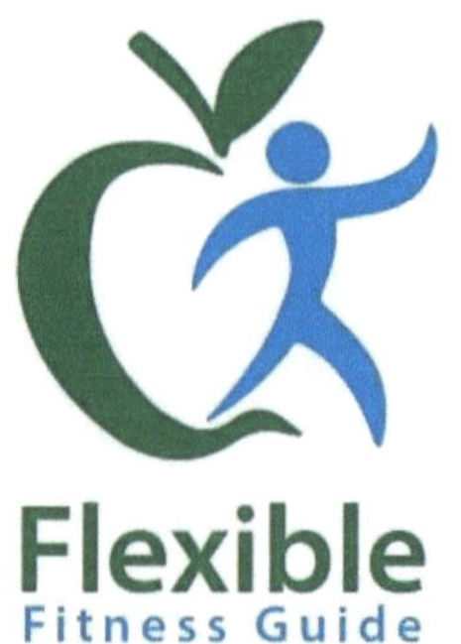

Total Daily Energy Expenditure

Let's continue to help Arnold achieve his fitness goals. We calculated Arnold's BMR to be 1,962 calories per day. We need to know Arnold's daily activity level in order to select the correct multiplier; this will allow us to convert Arnold's BMR to his TDEE.

Let's say Arnold works a desk job and lifts weights 4-5 times per week, putting Arnold in the "moderately active" category. 1.55 will be the appropriate multiplier in this example.

Arnold's TDEE

1,962 calories x 1.55 = 3,041 calories

What does this mean? Remember, your total daily energy expenditure tells you how many calories you burn on a given day, adjusted for your daily activity level. If Arnold were to consume 3,041 calories per day, his weight will remain stable.

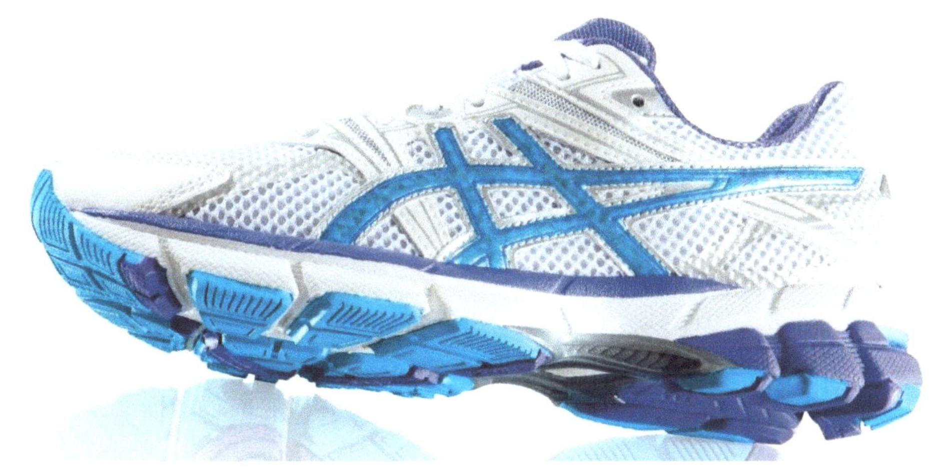

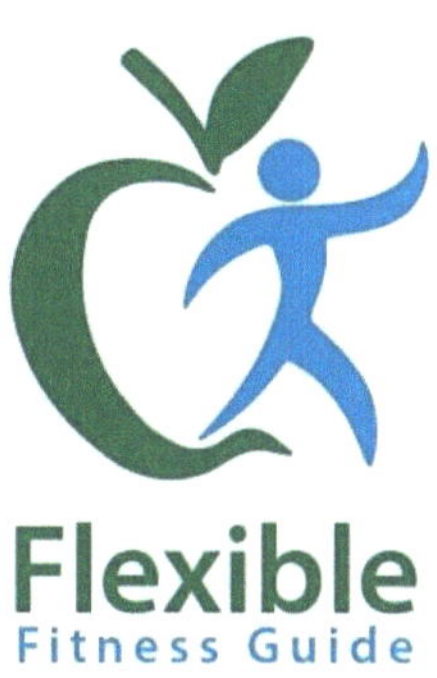

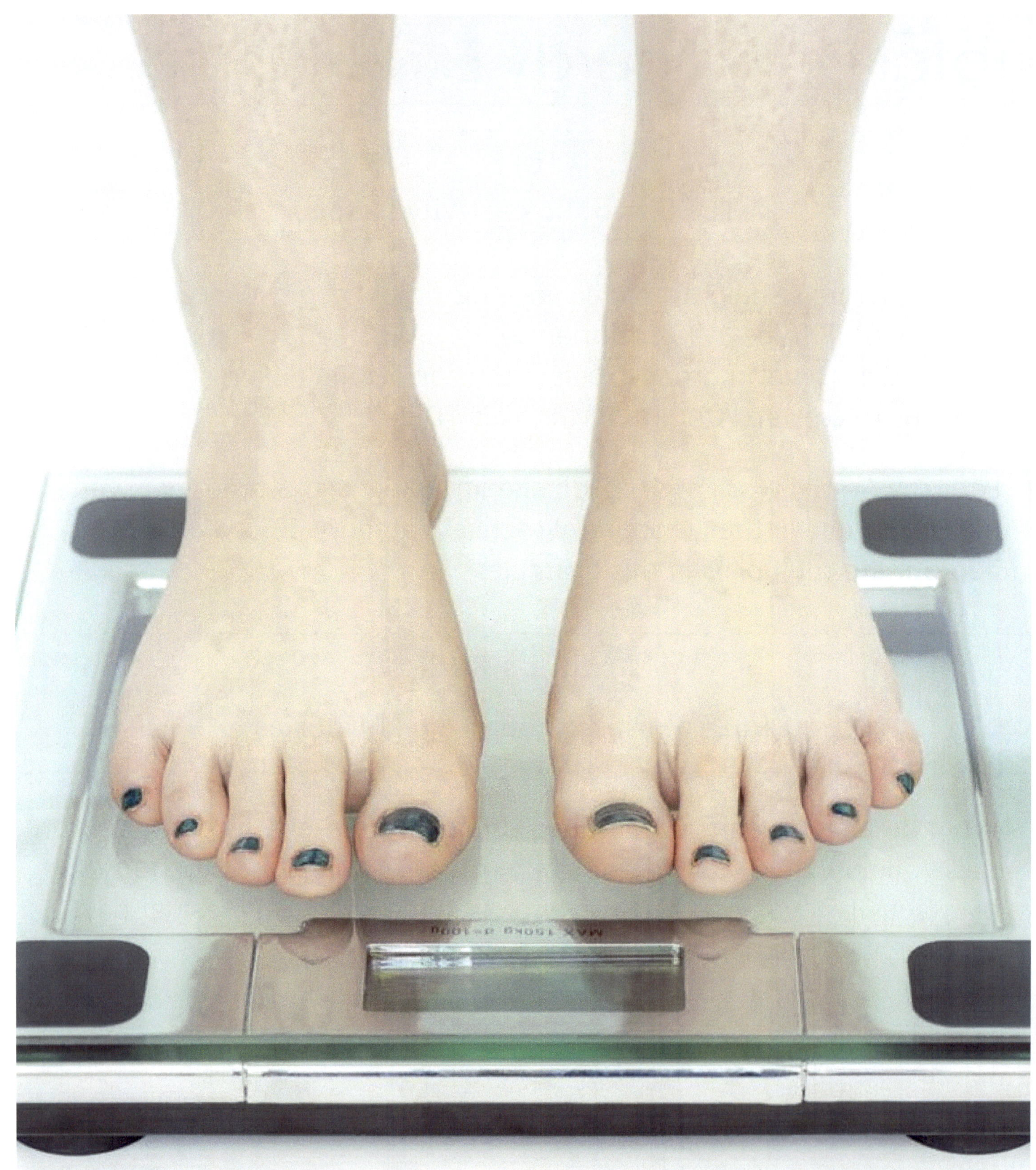

Chapter 2
Choosing a Diet Goal

Body Fat Percentage

With your TDEE in hand, you are equipped with a very powerful tool. You now have a marker with which you can determine the number of calories you need to consume to either gain or lose weight. BUT WAIT...do you want to gain, or lose weight? For some, there is an obvious answer; for others, it is not so clear.

For bodybuilders, there is a traditional method of cycling "cutting" (usually prior to beach season) and "bulking" (usually after beach season). We would like to bust this tradition and encourage a more sustainable methodology. The issue with cycling "cutting" with "bulking" is that usually they are taken to extremes; these extremes could lead to deleterious effects on one's health, lack of energy for peak gym performance, consumption of a mentally draining number of calories (too few or too many), an extremely high body fat percentage during bulking, and a variety of other complications.

The methodology we promote is staying under 12% body fat for men and under 20% for women year round. Contrast this with die-hard bodybuilders who achieve low single digit body fat during cutting season and, in some cases, bulk up to high teens and into the twenties during bulking season. These bodybuilders are not primarily concerned about their health and have the time on their hands to sustain these diets. By maintaining a healthy **body fat percentage** year round, you will remain energized, not have to constantly reconstruct your nutrition plan, avoid the mental taxation that comes along with extreme surpluses and deficits in caloric intake, and most importantly you will learn to be happy with your physique!

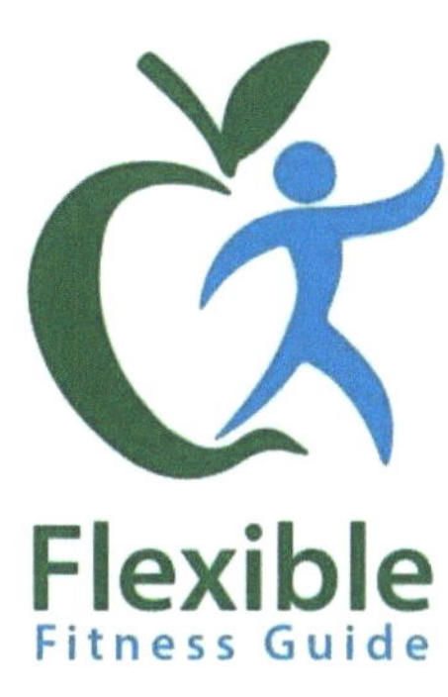

Body Fat Percentage

We need to measure your body fat percentage. If you are above 12% (men) or 20% (women), we recommend following through with Chapter 3 until you drop below that benchmark, or to your target body fat percentage. If you are already below your goal and are happy with your body fat percentage, we recommend jumping to chapter 4.

The formulas below will help you obtain a rough estimate on your body fat percentage. For a more accurate measurement, you are welcome to see a healthcare professional who is qualified to measure your body fat percentage for you.

For men, you will need two measurements: body weight and waist circumference.

1. Body weight
2. Waist circumference

For women, you will need five measurements.

1. Body weight
2. Waist circumference
3. Wrist circumference
4. Hip circumference
5. Forearm circumference

All of the measurements other than body weight (kilograms) will be in centimeters.

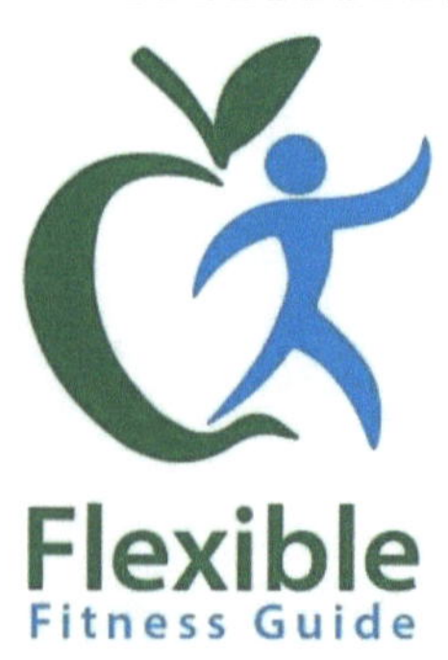

Body Fat Percentage

The best time to weigh yourself is first thing in the morning, upon waking up. Ideally, you should use the bathroom before stepping on the scale. Also, it is advised to weigh yourself with no clothing to avoid discrepancies. Note: LBM is lean body mass; BFW is body fat weight. We realize that these are lengthy calculations; please remain patient and do your best to get accurate results.

Body Fat Percentage for Men (kg, cm)

$$LBM = (weight\ x\ 2.38) + 94.42 - (waist\ size\ x\ 1.63)$$

$$BFW = (weight\ x\ 2.2) - LBM$$

$$Body\ Fat\ \% = (BFW\ x\ 100)/(weight\ x\ 2.2)$$

Body Fat Percentage for Women (kg, cm)

$$Factor\ 1 = (weight\ x\ 1.61) + 8.987$$

$$Factor\ 2 = wrist\ circumference/7.98$$

$$Factor\ 3 = waist\ circumference\ x\ 0.062$$

$$Factor\ 4 = hip\ circumference\ x\ 0.098$$

$$Factor\ 5 = forearm\ circumference\ x\ 0.171$$

$$LBM = Factor\ 1 + Factor\ 2 - Factor\ 3 - Factor\ 4 + Factor\ 5$$

$$BFW = (weight\ x\ 2.2) - LBM$$

$$Body\ Fat\ \% = (BFW\ x\ 100)/(weight\ x\ 2.2)$$

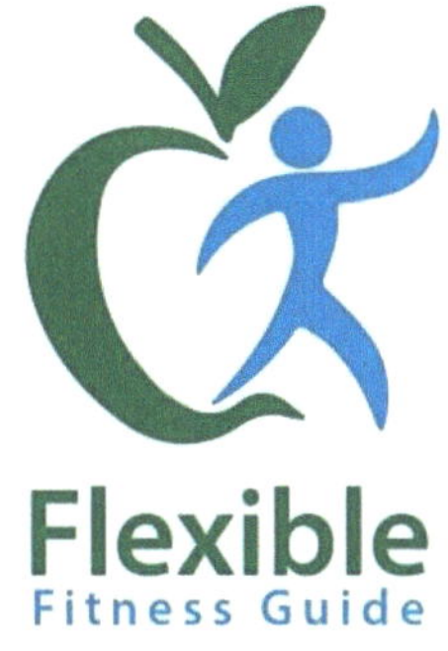

Body Fat Percentage

Once you have calculated your body fat percentage, simply refer to the below table to guide you in deciding whether you need to lose body fat or gain muscle mass. If you are near 12% (men)/20% (women), the choice is yours! You are always welcome to use a lower or higher benchmark. 12% (men) and 20% (women) is a reasonable benchmark that will allow you to look lean and not have to deal with an insufferable diet.

Current Body Fat Percentage	Goal
Under 12% (men) or 20% (women)	Gain mass
Over 12% (men) or 20% (women)	Lose fat

Let us continue tracking Arnold's fitness journey, as an example. He weighs 86.4 kilograms and has a waist size of 86 centimeters.

Body Fat Percentage for Men (kg, cm)

$$LBM = (86.4 \times 2.38) + 94.42 - (86 \times 1.63) = 159.87$$

$$BFW = (86.4 \times 2.2) - 159.87 = 30.21$$

$$Body\ Fat\ \% = (30.21 \times 100)/(86.4 \times 2.2) = 15.89\%$$

According to the above table, Arnold Columbu should follow a fat loss diet.

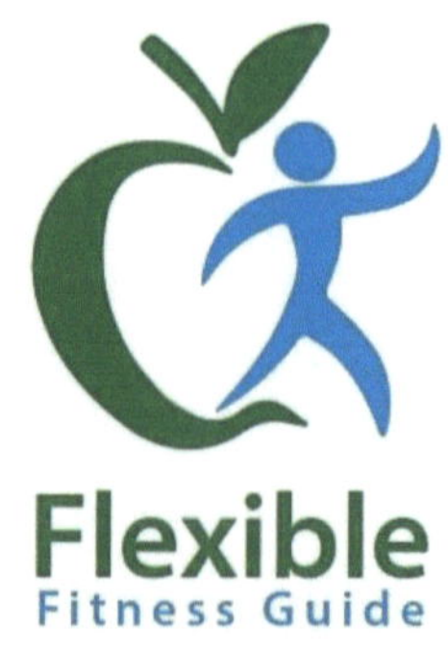

Body Fat Percentage

Remember, a continuous assessment of your progress is essential. When you are beginning your new diet, you should weigh yourself and calculate your body fat percentage at least once per week in case there are unforeseen fluctuations. As you become more adept at predicting changes in your body and handling your calories, you can use these measurements less and less frequently. The point is to hone in your skills as the manager of your own diet and of your own body. We're going for the whole "give a (wo)man a fish, feed him/her for a day; teach a (wo)man to fish, feed him/her for a lifetime" idea.

As your weight changes, you can modify your caloric intake and goal as needed.

For example, if Arnold followed a fat loss diet and got down to 10% body fat, he would then shift gears and begin to follow a mass gain diet. If managed properly, Arnold should maintain his body fat percentage while on his mass gain diet; however, if he notices his body fat percentage jump above 12%, he should consider switching back to the fat loss diet.

Please perform your body fat percentage calculations before proceeding. If you have come to the conclusion that you need a fat loss diet, please proceed to Chapter 3; if you have come to the conclusion that you need a mass gain diet, please proceed to Chapter 4 and refer back to Chapter 3 if you need advice for fat loss.

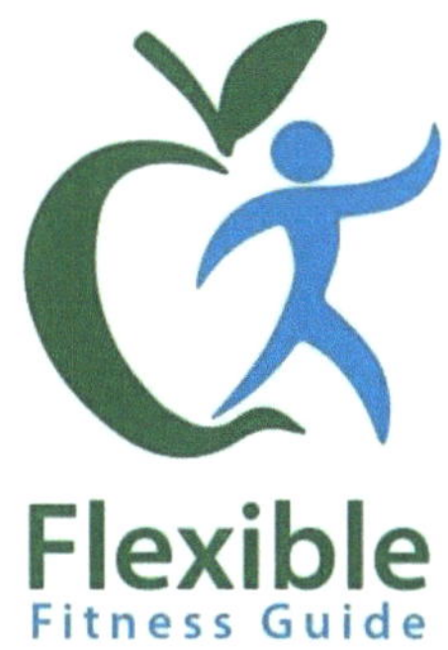

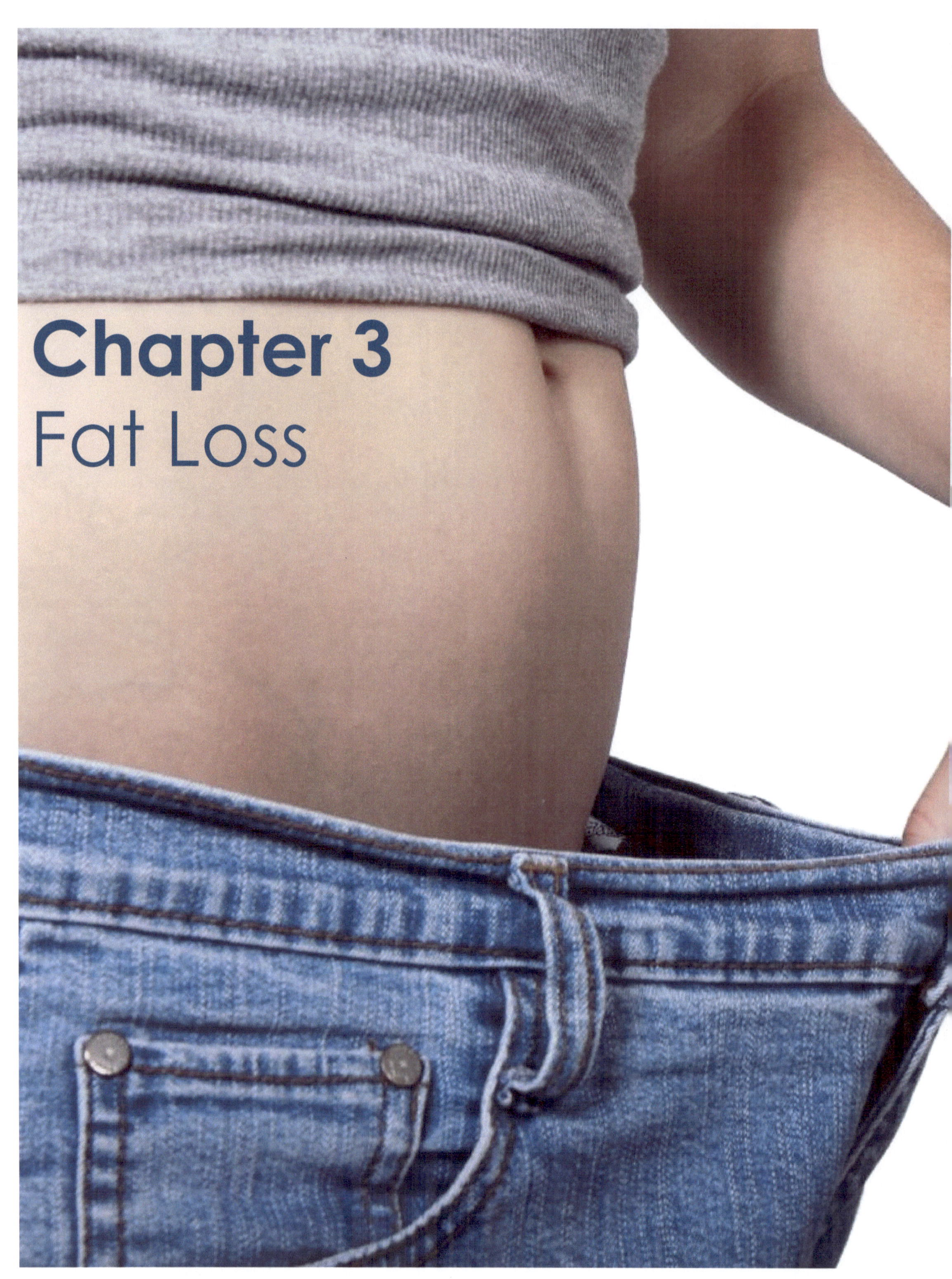
Chapter 3
Fat Loss

Caloric Deficit

For fat loss, you will need to enter a **caloric deficit. This means that the number of calories you consume must be less than the number of calories you expend on a daily basis.** So in Arnold's case, he must consume less than 3,041 calories per day to lose weight. Recall, 3,041 calories is the number that we calculated for Arnold's TDEE, or Total Daily Energy Expenditure, in Chapter 2.

Recognize that not all weight lost is in the form of fat. For most individuals, the average amount of fat that can be lost per week is 1 pound, plus or minus variations. For people with higher levels of fat stores, 1.5 to 2 pounds of fat will be easier to lose. For leaner individuals, even the 1 pound of pure fat may be difficult to lose.

Anything lost in excess of these ranges can be water weight, for instance. Individuals who have recently began exercising after leading a sedentary lifestyle or individuals who have made changes to their dietary habits can see hard-to-predict fluctuations in water weight.

Keeping in mind that the human body is a complex beast, we want to encourage you once again to seek long term success. If you are a week into your new plan and do not see results, do not be discouraged. Stick with it; if a month in you are still seeing absolutely no results, re-evaluate the precision with which you are following our guidelines and make adjustments.

"Stick with it"

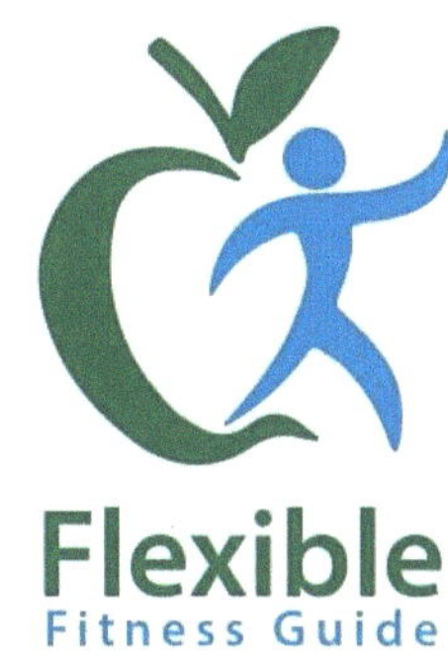

Caloric Deficit

Based on the body fat percentage you calculated in Chapter 3, please use the table below to pinpoint the caloric deficit that you should be attaining each day.

Current Body Fat Percentage	Calorie Deficit
6-10%	250
10-15%	500
Greater than 15%	750

The caloric deficit is higher for individuals with higher body fat percentages due to their excess fat stores. These individuals have high fat to muscle ratios. Muscle preservation is not as sensitive an issue for these individuals since the body prefers to burn fat when it is readily available.

As for individuals with lower body fat percentages, their caloric deficits are lower for the purpose of preserving muscle. These individuals have low fat to muscle ratios and have relatively less fat to lose. This makes muscle a more likely target for the body to burn compared to individuals with higher body fat percentages. The caloric deficit will be lower for these individuals to alleviate concerns of muscle loss.

Caloric Deficit

Let's see where Arnold stands on this spectrum. In the previous chapter, we determined that his body fat constitutes 15.89% of his total body weight. Since he falls in the third bracket, which includes individuals with body fat percentages greater than 15 %, he will have to subtract 750 calories from his TDEE for his fat loss diet.

Arnold's Calories for Fat Loss

$$\text{TDEE} - 750 = 3{,}041 - 750 = 2{,}291 \text{ calories}$$

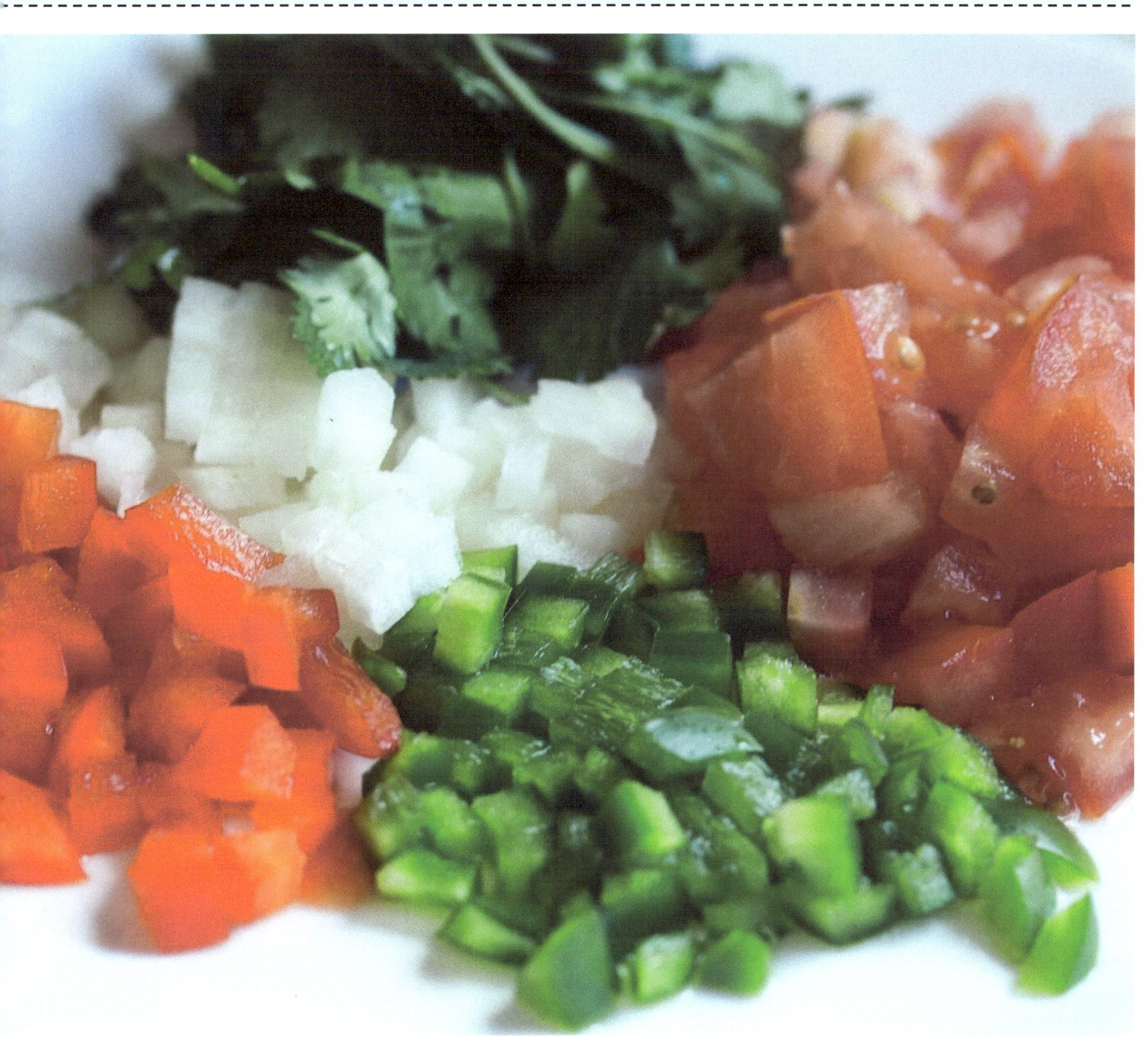

Macronutrients

Now that you have calculated your caloric intake for maximum, efficient fat loss, you must distribute these calories to their respective macronutrients. The three macronutrients you should be concerned with are protein, carbohydrates, and fat. Many people mistakenly believe that hitting their calorie goal for the day is sufficient. While it is true that you will still lose weight with the optimal caloric intake, the quality of the weight lost will not be up to par. Higher protein intake than you might expect will be necessary to maintain muscle mass. Please refer to the table below any time we reference the number of calories per gram of macronutrient.

Macronutrient	Calories Per Gram
Protein	4
Carbohydrate	4
Fat	9

Let us begin with protein intake. The percentage of total calories that protein takes up while on a fat loss diet is typically higher than when on a maintenance or mass gaining diet for the sake of muscle preservation. After much trial and error, we found that 2.86 grams of protein per kilogram of body weight is the ideal amount of protein to consume while on a fat loss diet. For Arnold, this equates to:

Arnold's Protein Intake
86.4 x 2.86 = 247 grams of protein

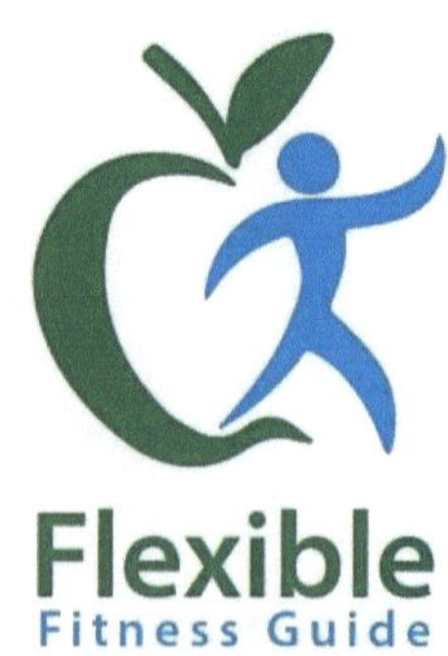

Macronutrients

Next, we recommend that 22% of total calories consumed be in the form of fat. Some people may go as high as 30%, but we prefer keeping it lower than 25% for the sake of saving room for carbohydrates. We feel that carbohydrates are an important source of energy for daily activities, especially workouts, given that they are ingested during appropriate time windows. Below is the calculation for Arnold's recommended fat intake. Remember, there are 9 calories per gram of fat that we ingest through our diet.

Arnold's Fat Intake

$$2{,}291 \times 0.22 \ (22\%) = 504 \text{ calories}$$

$$504 \text{ calories} \times 1 \text{ gram of fat}/9 \text{ calories} = 56 \text{ grams of fat}$$

Finally, let us examine carbohydrate intake. The remainder of your calories at this point will attributed to carbohydrates. Let's get started by calculating the number of calories that we have attributed to protein and fat thus far. In the previous calculation, you have calculated the calories that you should be consuming in fat per day. For Arnold, this is 504 calories attributable to fat intake. We know that Arnold is supposed to be consuming 247 grams of protein per day, and that there are 4 calories per gram of protein. Multiplying the two numbers together, we know that Arnold is consuming 988 calories in protein per day. Please complete this calculation for your personal diet plan.

Now, let's calculate how many calories of carbohydrates you should be consuming per day. We will simply use your allowed calorie consumption per day (calculated earlier in this chapter) and subtract the number of calories that you are to consume in protein and fat. Take a look at Arnold's calculations on the next page.

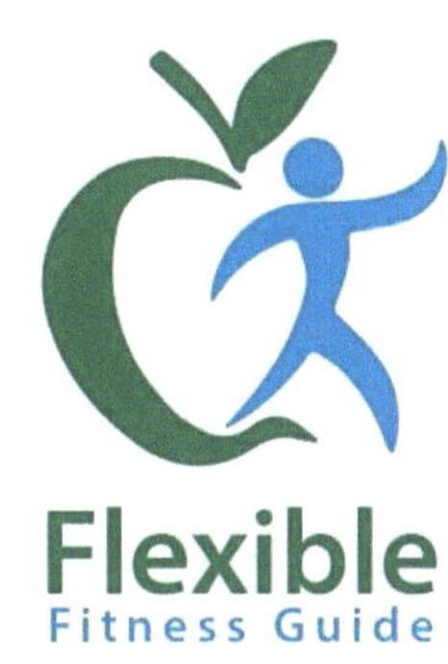

Macronutrients

> **Arnold's Remaining Calories**
> $$2{,}291 - 988 - 504 = 799 \text{ calories}$$

So, Arnold will be consuming 799 calories in carbohydrates per day while on his fat loss diet. Considering 4 calories per gram of carbohydrate, we use the example below to demonstrate how many grams of carbohydrates Arnold will be consuming per day.

> **Arnold's Carbohydrate Intake**
> $$799 \text{ calories} \times 1 \text{ gram}/4 \text{ calories} = 200 \text{ grams of carbohydrates}$$

Please take the time to build yourself a table like the one below to summarize your daily intake allowances. Below is Arnold's diet plan.

Macronutrient	Calculation	Intake (grams)	Intake (calories)
Protein	Body weight x 2.86	247	988
Fat	22% of calories	56	504
Carbohydrates	Remainder of calories	200	799
Total	Sum of macronutrients	503	2,291

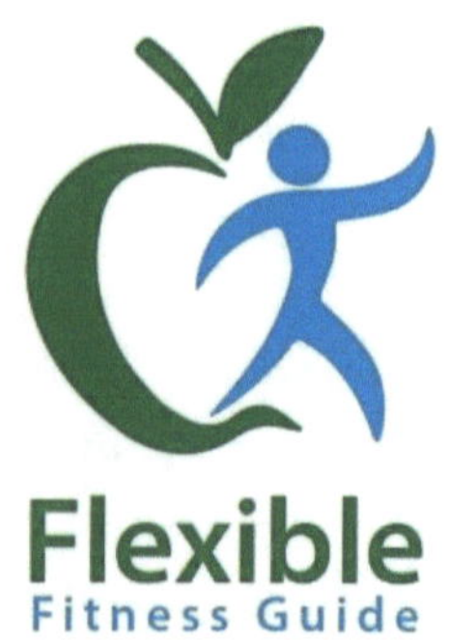

Meal Timing

Now that we have covered our macronutrients, let us talk a little bit about **nutrient timing and meal frequency**. We recommend an average of 3 hours between meals to provide your muscles with a steady source of protein that will prevent muscle breakdown.

Carbohydrate intake is the most important macronutrient regarding the timing of your consumption. It is preferred to split your carbohydrate intake between two or three meals. If you exercise in the morning, split it between two meals; if you exercise at a different time, split it between three meals.

Your first meal of the day (breakfast) should include a significant amount of carbohydrates order to fuel yourself to perform your daily activities. Another meal, about 2-3 hours before you exercise, should include the majority of carbohydrates to fuel your workout. If you work out in the morning, simply eat a lot of carbohydrates before going to the gym, essentially combining the recommended carbohydrate consumption of the two mentioned meals into one. The final meal containing a significant amount of carbohydrates should be your post-workout meal to replenish your muscles glycogen stores.

Meal	Carbohydrate Intake (% of total carbohydrates)
Breakfast (first meal of the day)	20%
Pre-workout (2 hours before workout)	35%
Post-Workout (2 hours after workout)	35%
Remainder of meals	10%

Meal Timing

As for the types of carbohydrates to consume, we typically recommend low glycemic index, slow digesting carbohydrates (see Sample Foods chapter) for most meals (breakfast, pre-workout, and post-workout). Put simply, this means that instead of consuming candy bars and soda, we choose to consume things like whole grain rice or whole wheat bread, particularly for breakfast and pre-workout. For post-workout, fast digesting carbohydrates like ice cream or fruit juice are more acceptable. Vegetables are another source of nutrient-rich carbohydrates that will help contribute to your overall health.

As for fat intake, we recommend keeping it as low as possible during the high-carbohydrate meals: breakfast, pre-workout, and post-workout. The remainder of the fat should be spread as evenly as possible across the remaining low-carbohydrate meals. Protein should be split evenly across all of your daily meals. See the below table for a sample split of Arnold's macronutrients. This should be a good guide to help you with your split if any of the information thus far is unclear.

Meal	Protein	Carbohydrate	Fat
Breakfast	1/6 of total = 41 grams	18.5% = 37 grams	10-11% = 6 grams
Lunch	1/6 of total = 41 grams	3% = 6 grams	35-36% = 20 grams
Pre-Workout	1/6 of total = 41 grams	43.5% = 87 grams	5-6% = 3 grams
During Workout	1/6 of total = 41 grams	0% = 0 grams	3-4% = 2 grams
Post-Workout	1/6 of total = 41 grams	31% = 62 grams	0% = 0 grams
Dinner	1/6 of total = 41 grams	4% = 8 grams	44-45% = 25 grams
Total	246 grams	200 grams	56 grams

Meal Timing

Keep in mind that the percentages in the table are for the purpose of guidance. They are not in set in stone and if you are not accurate down to the last gram, you will still make progress and lose fat! Do not stress; a couple of grams here or there will not make or break you. That is not encouragement to deviate far from the guidelines, but please do not panic over every detail. Remember, if you are making the progress that you hope to make, then you are succeeding.

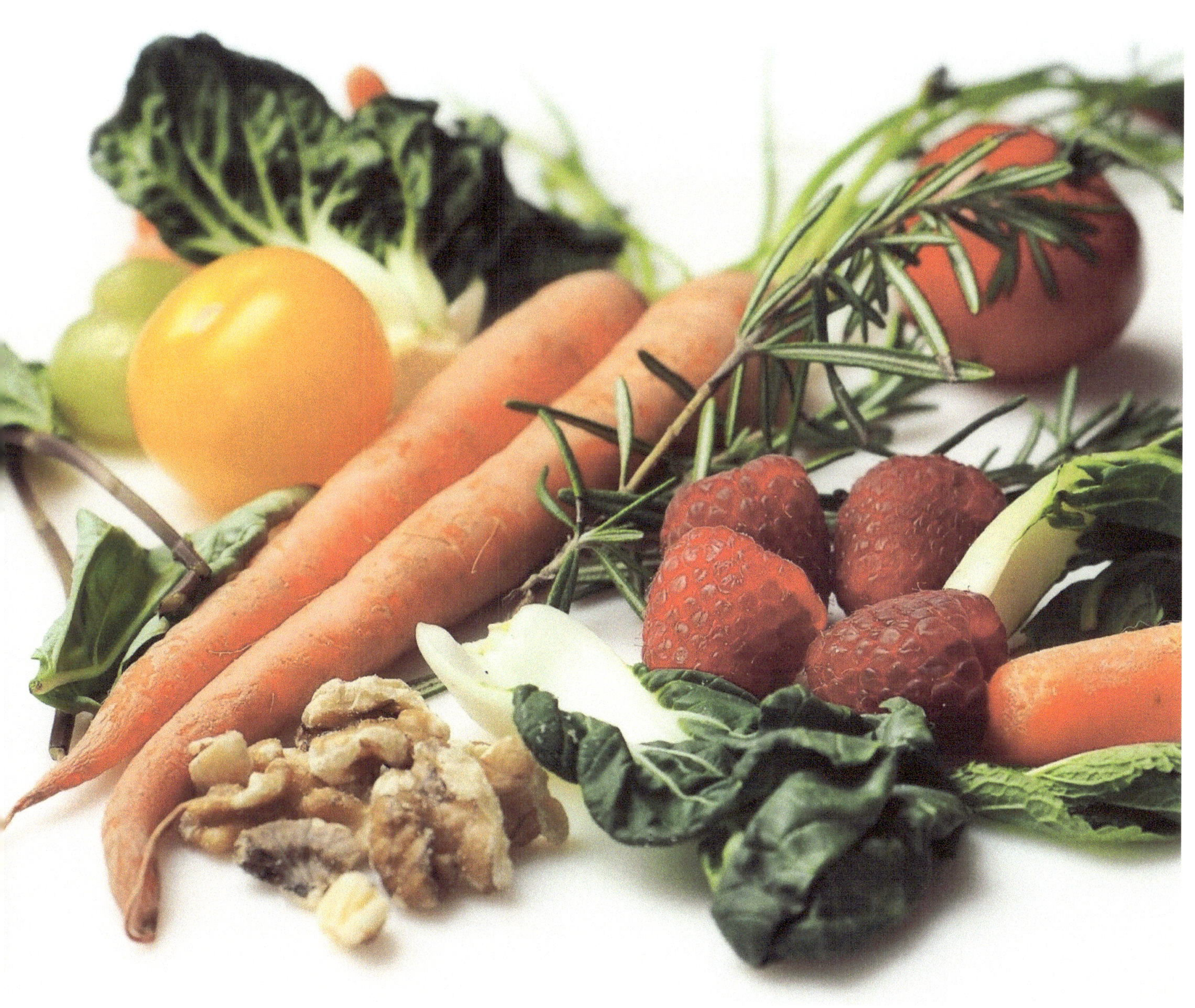

Refeed Day

Now to the fun part of the fat loss diet: the refeed day. You will bump your calories up to equal your TDEE. For instance, Arnold will be consuming 3,041 calories on a refeed day. In short, this will replenish your muscle's glycogen stores and manipulate your hormones to provide you with the physiological and psychological energy your need to tackle the upcoming week's schedule. Please refer to the table below in order to figure out how often you should have a refeed day.

Body Fat Percentage	Frequency
6-10%	2 refeed days per week
10-15%	1 refeed day per week
>15%	1 refeed day every two weeks

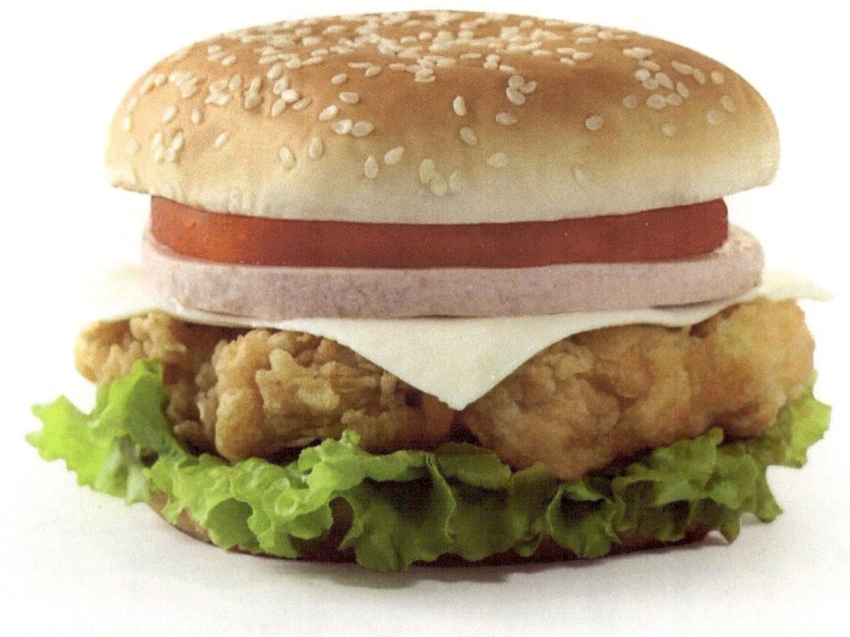

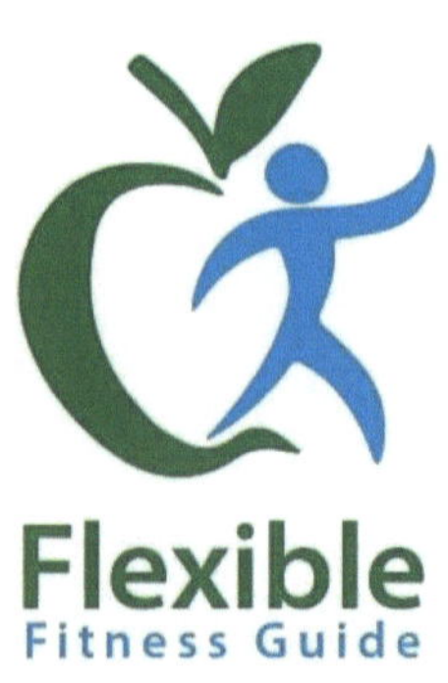

Refeed Day

We recommend that you schedule your refeed days for when you have tough workouts, such as on leg day. Some quick hit points to consider when structuring your refeed days:

1. Bring your calories up to maintenance (TDEE)
2. Reduce protein intake to 1 gram per pound of body weight
3. Double your carbohydrate intake (WOOHOO!)
4. The rest of your calories will come from fats

Using Arnold as an example, here is how his macronutrients will look on his refeed day (at 3,041 calories):

Macronutrient	Calculation	Intake (grams)	Intake (calories)
Protein	Body weight x 2.2	190	760
Carbohydrates	Regular intake x 2	400	1,600
Fat	Remainder of calories	76	681
Total	Sum of macronutrients	666	3,041

For sample fat loss meal plans, refer to the Sample Meal Plans chapter. You are now equipped with your entire calorie and macronutrient count. This is a powerful tool — we know the math was hard, but you now have the power to become SHREDDED!

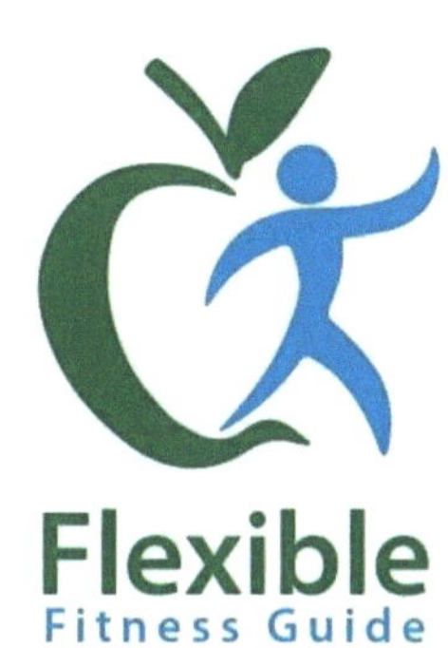

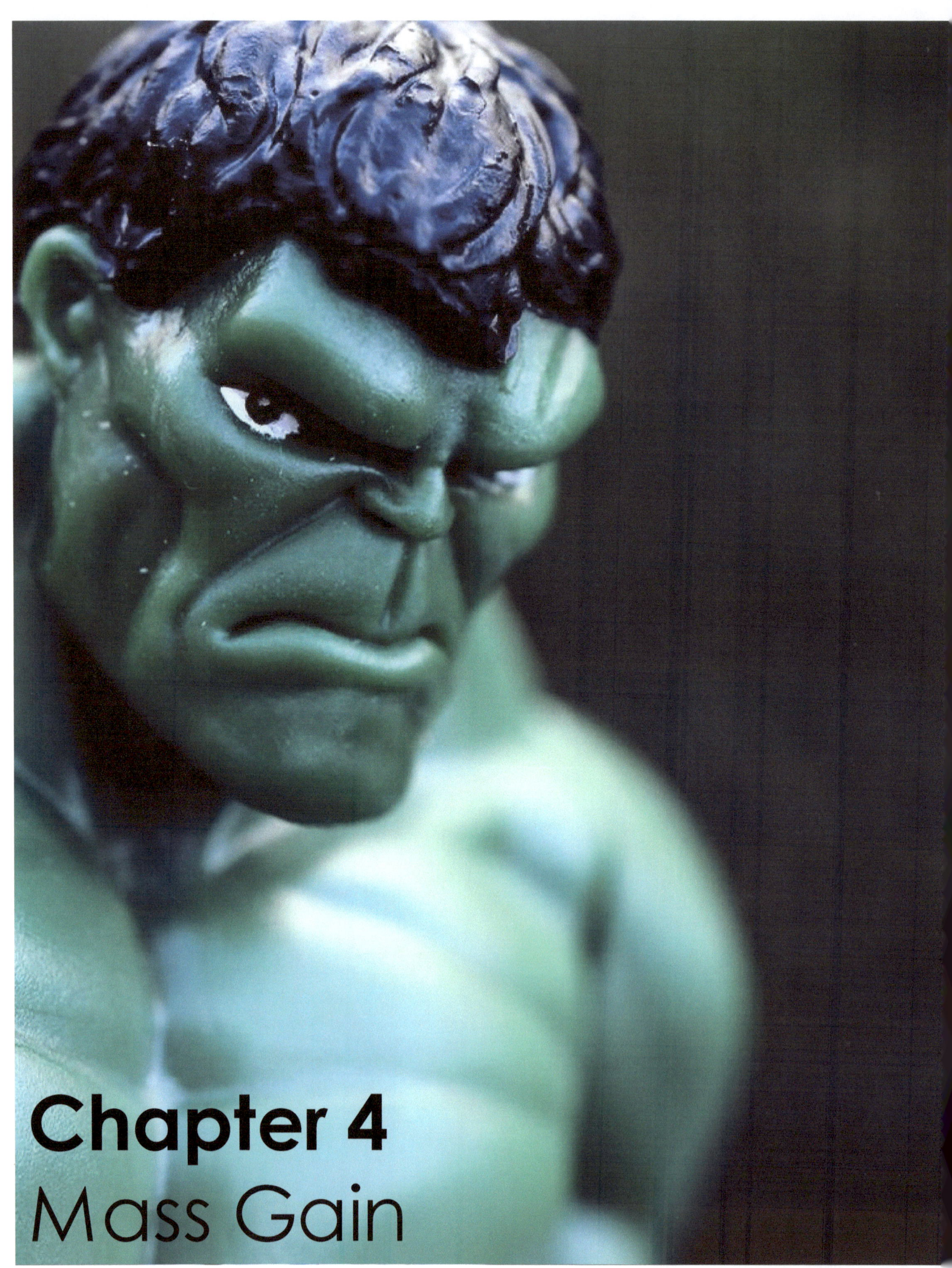

Chapter 4
Mass Gain

Caloric Surplus

To gain mass, you will need to consume more calories than you expend; this is referred to as a calorie surplus. So in Arnold's case, he must consume more than 3,041 calories (his TDEE) per day to gain weight.

Many people mistake the green light granted to enter a calorie surplus for a green light to eat anything and everything in sight. Do not fall for this trap. Please do not engage in chronic "dirty bulking," or eating any food you please. You do not want to put on the excess fat that comes with an "anything goes" diet; this will lead to the need for a fat loss diet much more quickly than you hope for. To be clear, our goal is to help you sustain a healthy lifestyle. Having to frequently switch back to a fat loss diet and having to recalculate your consumption is not conducive to a sustainable and enjoyable fitness lifestyle. Follow the road to success!

We recommend adding 500 calories as a surplus to your TDEE. For instance, Arnold's TDEE is 3,041 calories. Thus, he will consume 3,541 calories for his mass gain diet.

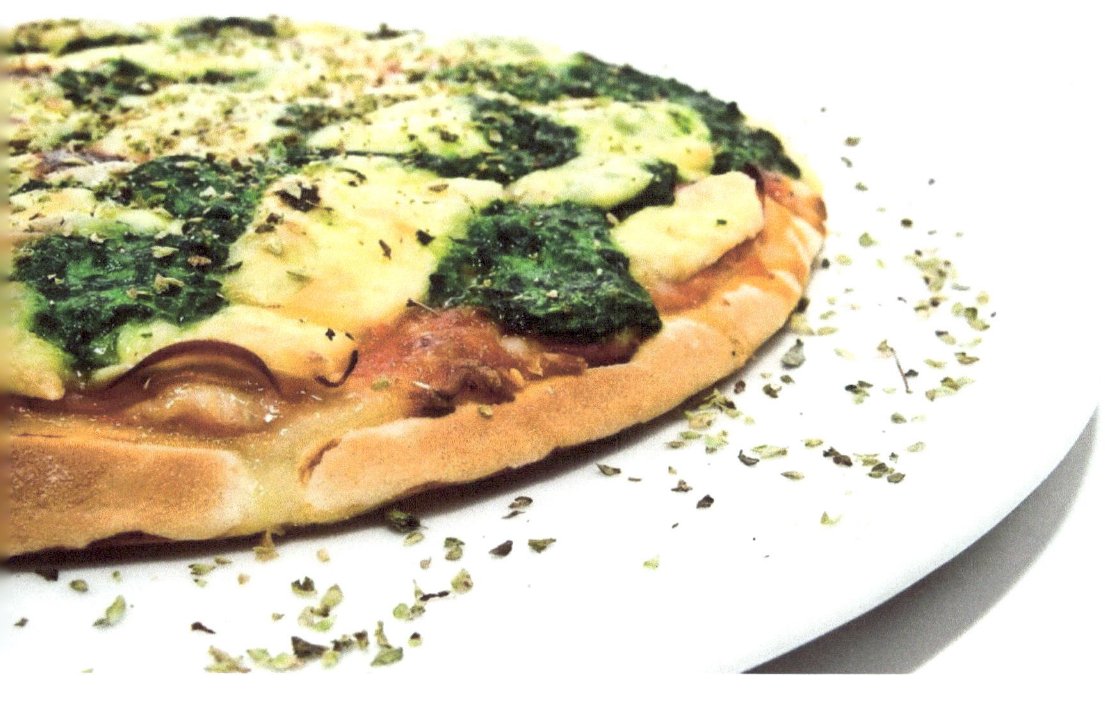

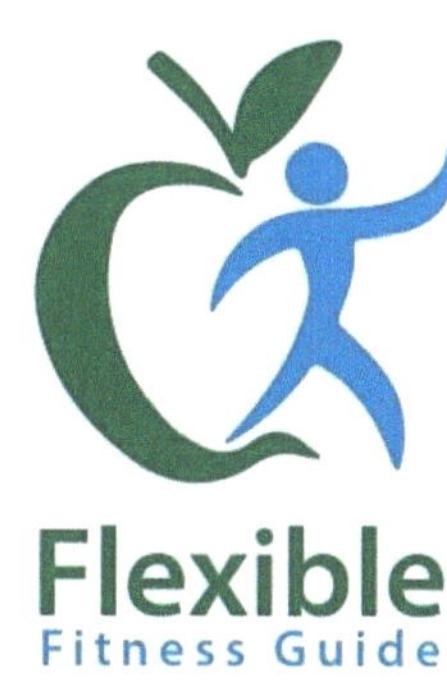

Calorie Distribution

Now that you have calculated your caloric intake for maximum, efficient mass gain, you must distribute these calories to their respective macronutrients. The three macronutrients you should be concerned with are protein, carbohydrates, and fat. To optimize the weight that you are gaining (muscle vs. fat), we will focus on the ratios of these macronutrients. Please refer to the table below any time we reference the number of calories per gram of macronutrient.

Macronutrient	Calories Per Gram
Protein	4
Carbohydrate	4
Fat	9

Let's start with protein. The percentage of total calories that protein takes up while on a mass gaining diet is typically lower than when on a fat loss diet. The abundance of calories you will be consuming allows your body to rely on more efficient sources of energy than protein. It is generally accepted that 2.2 grams per kilogram of body weight is sufficient to add muscle mass. Let's see how many grams of protein Arnold will be consuming on his mass gaining diet. Arnold weighs 86.4 kilograms and will consume 2.2 grams of protein per kilogram of bodyweight.

Arnold's Protein Intake

$$86.4 \text{ kilograms} \times \frac{2.2 \text{ grams of protein}}{\text{kilogram}} = 190 \text{ grams of protein}$$

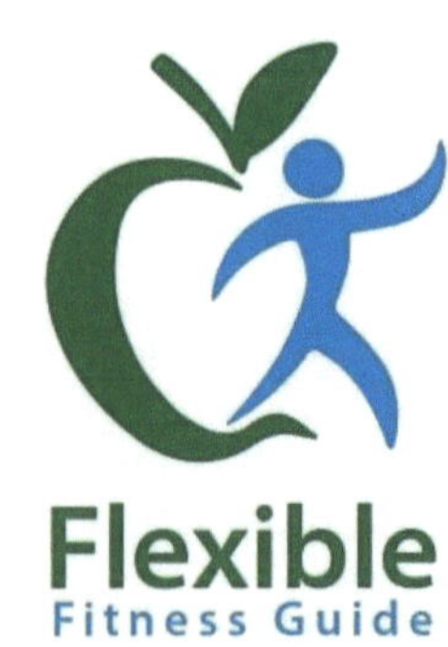

Calorie Distribution

Moving on to fat intake, we recommend 30% of total calories come from fat. A lower fat intake would be ideal, but it can be difficult to consume the high daily requirements of calories without consuming more fat. Feel free to adjust this figure to anywhere between 25-35%. We will use the average of the two extremes for our example.

Arnold's Fat Intake

$$3{,}541 \text{ calories} \times 0.30 = 1{,}062 \text{ calories}$$

$$1{,}062 \text{ calories} \times \frac{1 \text{ gram of fat}}{9 \text{ calories}} = 118 \text{ grams of fat}$$

That leaves us with the final macronutrient: the carbohydrate. The remainder of your calories to this point should be in the form of carbohydrates. So far, we know that Arnold is consuming 190 grams of protein (or 760 calories) and 118 grams of fat (or 1,062 calories). Subtracting the two from the 3,541 calories that Arnold will be consuming per day, we know that he must consume 1,719 calories in the form of carbohydrates (or 430 grams). Please remember to refer to the table earlier in this chapter for calories per gram of macronutrient. Please complete these calculations for your personal diet plan.

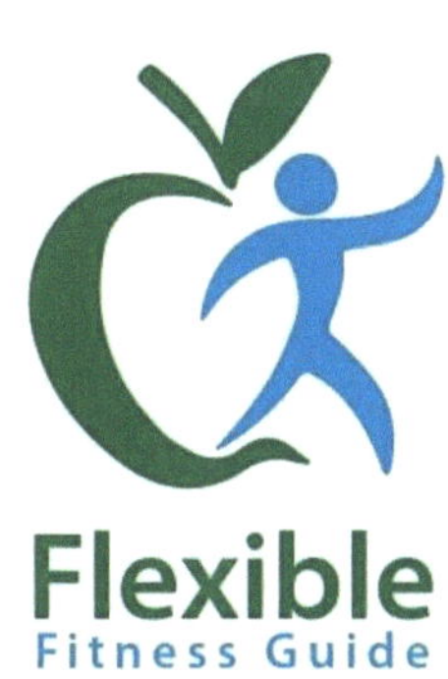

Calorie Distribution

To summarize, here is a table containing the information on the macronutrient breakdown (using Arnold as an example, of course). Please construct a similar table for your personal diet plan.

Macronutrient	Calculation	Intake (grams)	Intake (calories)
Protein	Body weight x 2.2	190	760
Fat	30% of calories	118	1,062
Carbohydrates	Remainder of calories	430	1,719
Total	Sum of macronutrients	738	3,541

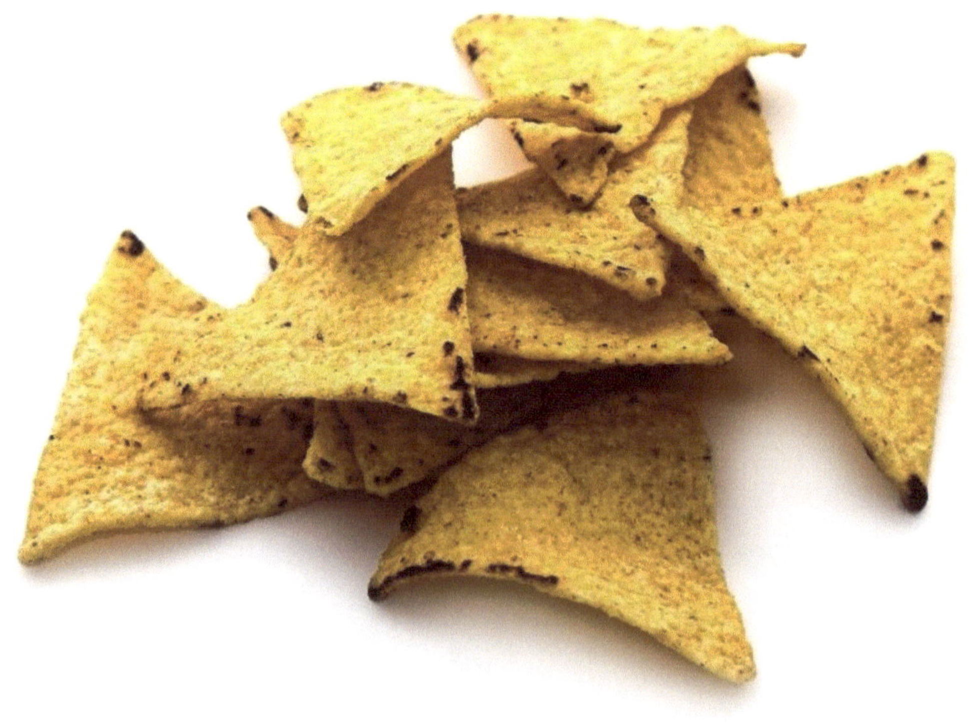

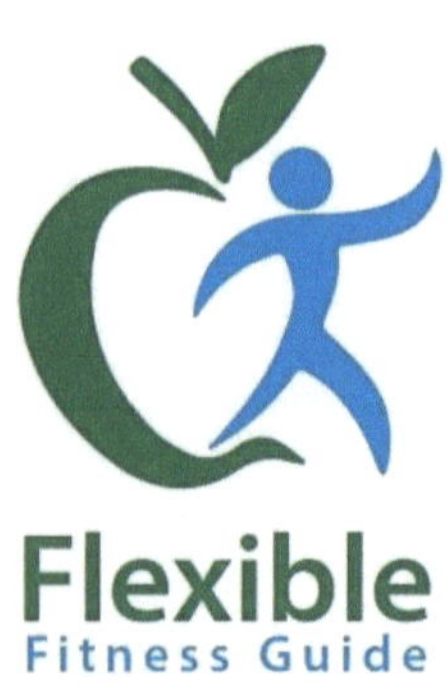

Meal Timing

Now that we have covered our macronutrients, let us talk a little bit about nutrient timing and meal frequency. We recommend an average of 3-5 hours between meals to provide your muscles with a steady source of protein that will prevent muscle breakdown.

During a mass gaining diet, meal timing is not as important as it is during a fat loss diet. We prefer a reasonable approach and break our meals down to 3-5 daily meals while on a mass gaining diet. This keeps us satiated and energized throughout the day in order to maximize our effort in the gym and optimize muscle growth.

The distribution of macronutrients throughout the day will also not be an extremely critical factor. We take advantage of the excess calories and the ability our bodies have to gain mass to follow an IIFYM approach during this time. IIFYM is an acronym for "if it fits your macros." Essentially, if a meal you'd like to eat is allowed based on your diet plan, eat it! Remember though, do not take this as a pass to eat all of the junk food that you can stomach. Keep it healthy overall and feel free to fit in some of your favorite foods here and there; you earned it!

For sample mass gain meal plans, refer to the Sample Meal Plans chapter. You are now equipped with your entire calorie and macronutrient count. This is a powerful tool – we know the math was hard, but you now have the power to become HUGE!

Chapter 5
Sample Meal Plans

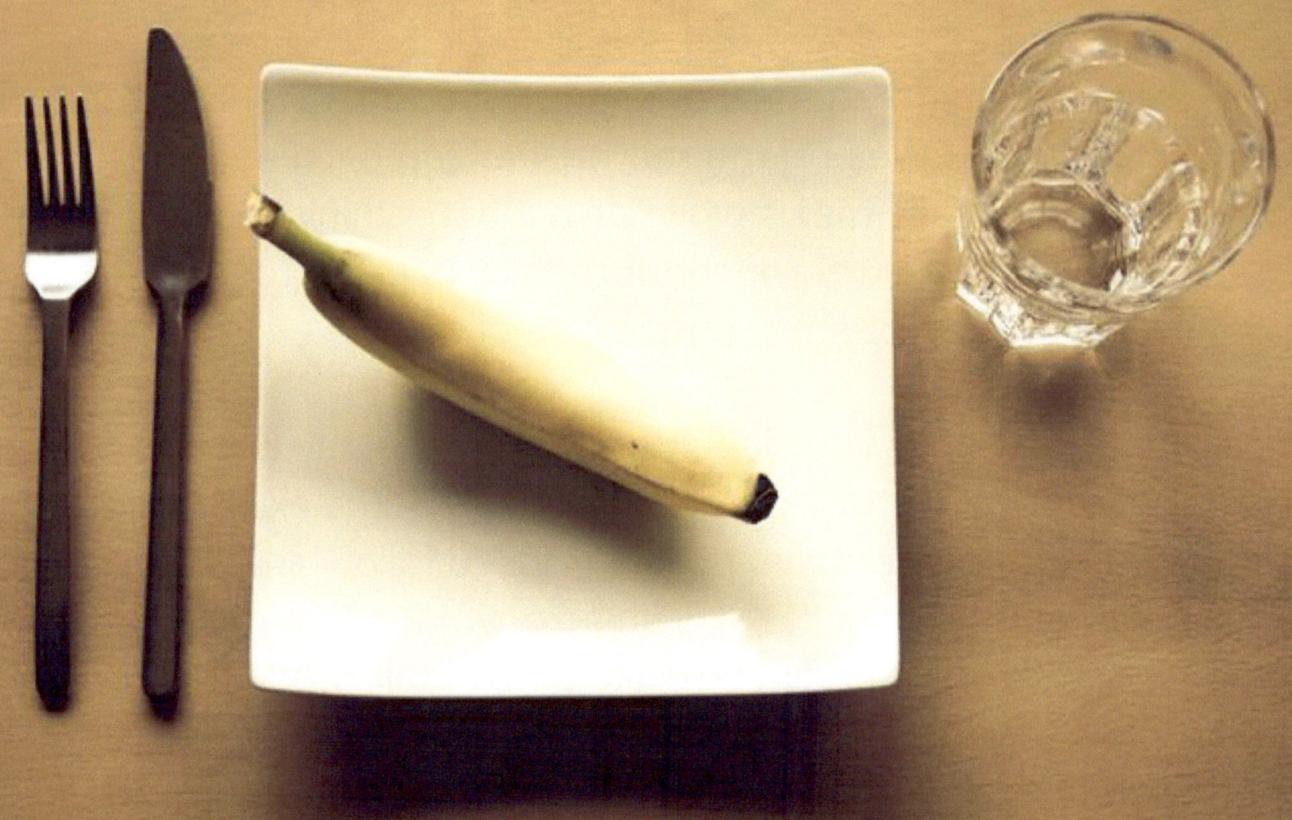

Sample Fat Loss Meal Plan

Based on Arnold Columbu's caloric deficit (2,291 calories) and macronutrient ratios, a sample fat loss meal plan he would set for himself might be as follows:

Macronutrient	Calculation	Intake
Protein	Body weight x 2.86	247 grams
Carbohydrate	Remainder of calories after protein and fat are calculated	200 grams
Fat	22% of total calories	56 grams

The table on the next page is a template to use as a guideline. Try to follow it as much as possible, but do not stress if your numbers do not perfectly match up. However, do keep the macronutrient guidelines from the Fat Loss chapter in mind when determining the distribution of your calories. Notice the high carbohydrate intake for breakfast and directly before and after workouts. Of course, the tables in this chapter use our example of Arnold Columbu throughout; please construct your tables according to the caloric requirements you calculated for yourself using the information in previous chapters.

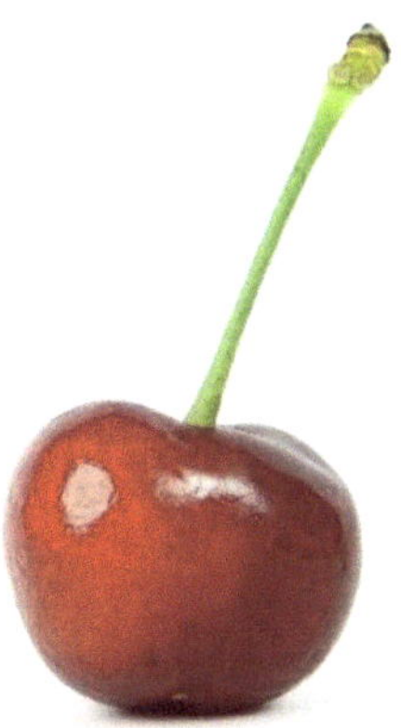

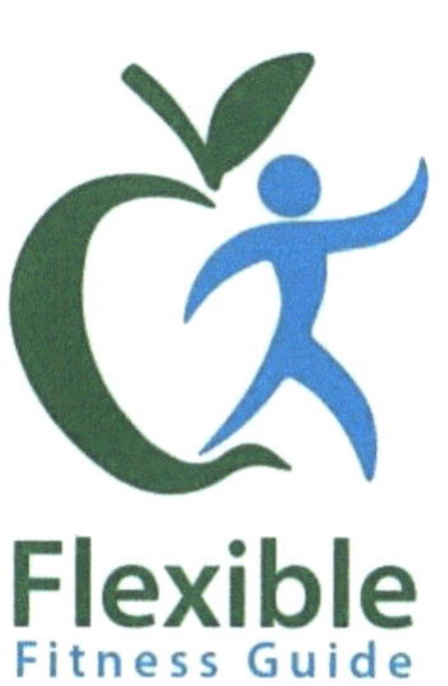

Sample Fat Loss Meal Plan

Meal	Food	Protein	Carbs	Fat
Breakfast	• 10 egg whites • ½ oz. shredded Cheddar cheese • 1 slice whole wheat bread • 1 tbsp. apple butter	42g	35g	5g
Lunch	• 6 oz. chicken breast • 2 tsp. olive oil • 1 cup broccoli	43g	6g	17g
Pre-Workout	• 1 cup oats (measure dry) • 1 banana • 1 scoop whey protein	36g	85g	6g
During Workout	• 1 scoop whey protein	27g	0g	2g
Post-Workout	• 8 oz. tilapia • 1.25 cup brown rice (measure cooked) • 1 cup asparagus	54g	61g	6g
Dinner	• 1 London Broil Steak • ½ cup Brussel sprouts	46g	4g	28g
Total	2,332 calories	248g	191g	64g

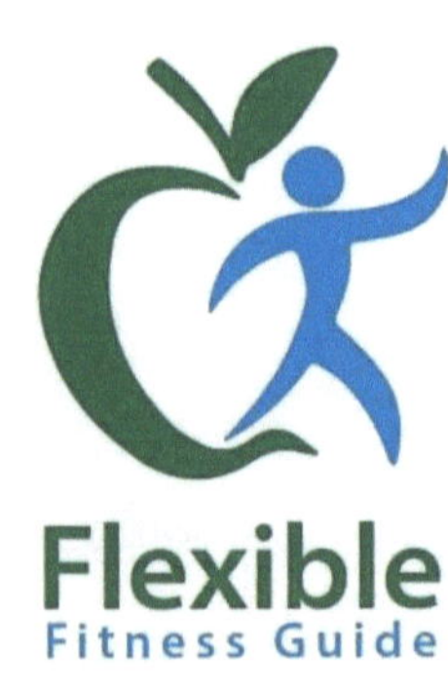

Sample Fat Loss Refeed Day

Based on Arnold's maintenance calories (3,041 calories) and macronutrient ratios, a sample refeed day meal plan that he would set for himself might be as follows:

Macronutrient	Calculation	Intake
Protein	Body weight (kg) x 2.2	190 grams
Carbohydrate	Double intake of fat loss days	400 grams
Fat	Remainder of calories	76 grams

The below table is a template to use as a guideline. Try to follow it as much as possible, but do not stress if your numbers do not perfectly match up.

Meal	Food	Protein	Carbs	Fat
Breakfast	• 1 wheat bagel • 2 tbsp. fat free cream cheese • ½ scoop whey protein • ½ cup orange juice	30g	74g	4g
Lunch	• 4 oz. chicken breast • 1½ tbsp. olive oil • 2 cups broccoli	32g	12g	20g
Pre-Workout	• 4 cups white rice (measure cooked) • ½ scoop whey protein	29g	181g	3g
During Workout	• 1 scoop whey protein	24g	2g	2g
Post-Workout	• 4 oz. chicken breast • 2 cups white rice (measure cooked)	38g	123g	2g
Dinner	• 8 oz. ground turkey • 2 tbsp. olive oil • 1 cup Brussel sprouts	35g	8g	41g
Total	3,000 calories	188g	400g	72g

Sample Mass Gain Meal Plan

Based on Arnold's maintenance calories (3,041 calories) and macronutrient ratios, a sample mass gain meal plan he would set for himself might be as follows:

Macronutrient	Calculation	Intake
Protein	Body weight x 2.2	190 grams
Carbohydrate	Remainder of calories after protein and fat are calculated	430 grams
Fat	30% of total calories	118 grams

The below table is just a template to use as a guideline. Try to follow it as much as possible, but do not stress if your numbers do not perfectly match up.

Meal	Food	Protein	Carbs	Fat
Breakfast	• 1 wheat bagel • 2 eggs • 2 slices turkey bacon • ½ cup orange juice	30g	71g	18g
Lunch	• 5 oz. sirloin steak • 1 ½ cups brown rice (measure cooked) • 2 tsp. olive oil	36g	67g	18g
Pre-Workout	• 1 cup oats (measure dry) • 1 cup skim milk • 1 tbsp. butter	31g	69g	18g
During Workout	• 2 cups chocolate milk (full fat)	24g	78g	25g
Post-Workout	• 6 oz. ground chicken • 1 ¾ cups white rice (measure cooked)	36g	78g	18g
Dinner	• 5 oz. sirloin steak • 1 ½ cups brown rice • 2 tsp. olive oil	36g	67g	18g
Total	3,527 calories	193g	430g	115g

Recommended Food Sources

Protein

Tilapia

Cod

Tuna

Egg Whites

Chicken Breast

93% Lean Ground Beef

Whey Protein

Carbohydrates

Oatmeal

Sweet Potatoes

Potatoes (when on a mass gain diet)

Brown Rice

White Rice (limit to pre- and post-workout)

Whole Grain Breads

Fruits

Vegetables

Fats

Olive Oil

Grass Fed Butter

Nuts (almonds, cashews, pecans, walnuts)

Natural Peanut Butter

Almond Butter

The easiest way to find out if the foods you desire fit within your macronutrient counts is to use a nutritional value search tool. Our favorite website that contains a vast database of most foods is www.calorieking.com.

There are also mobile cell phone applications that help you track your goals and keep your macronutrient counts in check. The best application out there is LifeSum or MyFitnessPal. We have no financial incentive to recommend any of the websites or applications on this page.

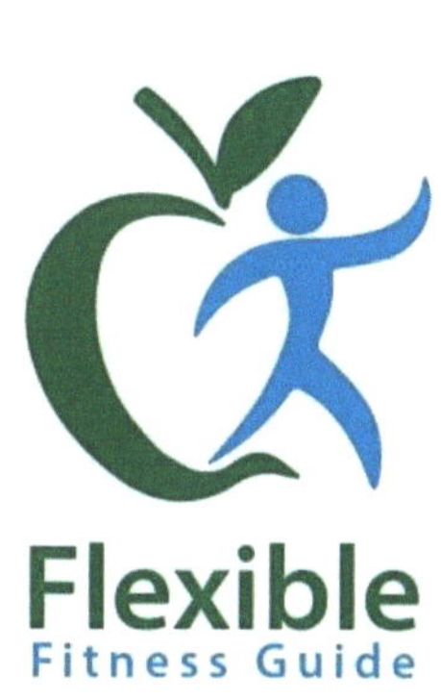

Chapter 6
Miscellaneous

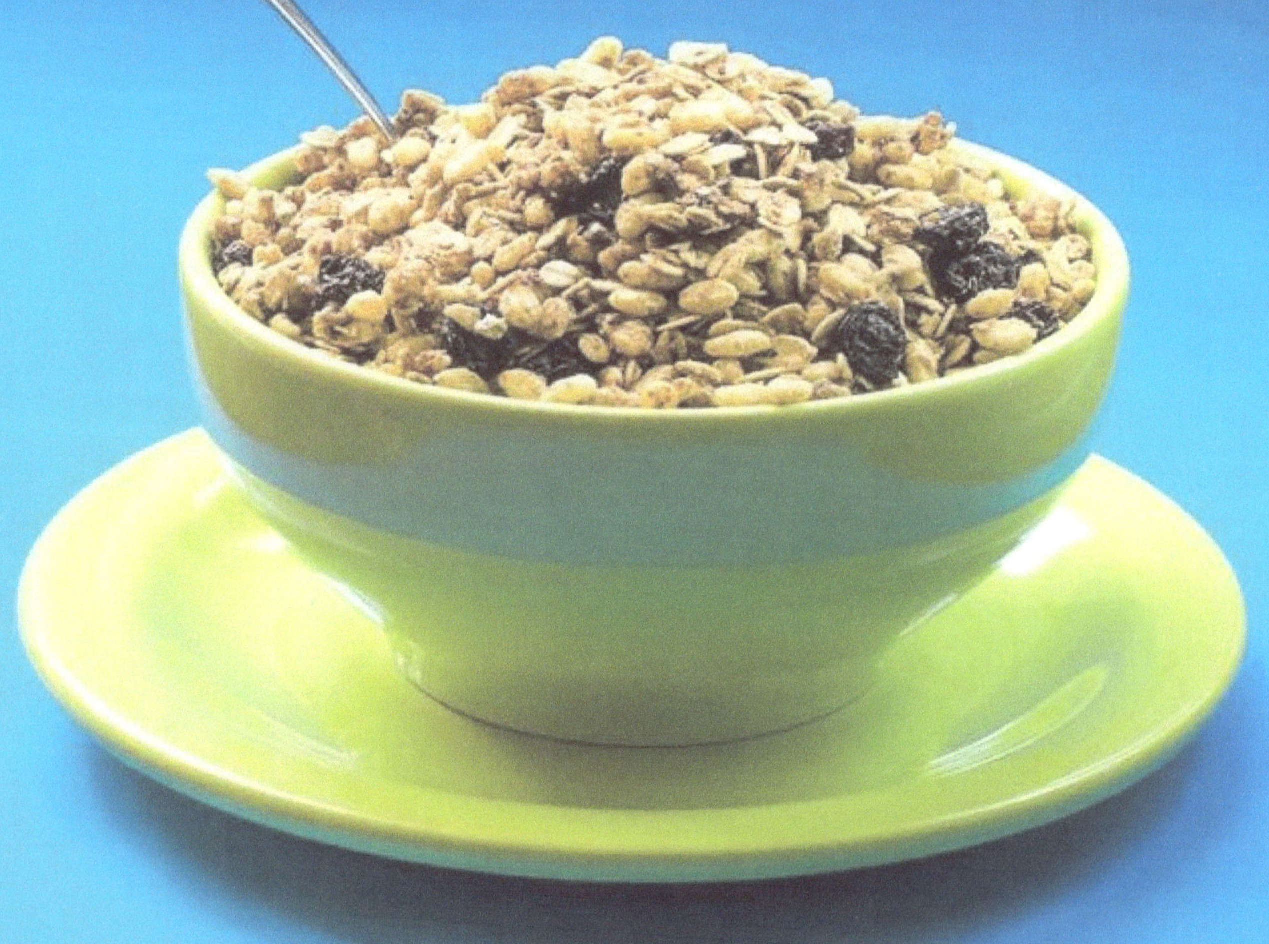

Water Intake

Now that we have you set up with the optimal caloric intake and helped you calculate your macronutrient ratios, we must turn to the issue of water intake. Many people often neglect water intake, which is in and of itself very critical to the success of any athlete. Dehydration can lead to cramping, nausea, and fatigue.

The minimum amount of water any person should intake on a given day is 1 gallon. For those of you doing heavy cardio workouts and sweating excessively, you should increase your intake to 1.5 gallons. This will vary from person to person, however, as we all have different body sizes. A general rule of thumb that if you weigh 150 pounds or less, you should drink 1 gallon of water every day. For people weighing over 150 pounds, add a glass (8 fl. oz.) of water for every 10 pounds you weigh over the 150 pounds. For example, if you weigh 200 pounds, that would equate to 1 gallon + 40 fl. oz., which is around 1.3 gallons of water.

As for the source of water intake, do not count every fluid in your count. If you drink coffee, soda, milk, juice or any other fluid, that does not count towards your daily intake. It may be difficult at first to hit your daily goal, but overtime you will adapt to the high fluid intake. **This system of only counting pure water will help you reduce the amount of high sugar beverages that you may otherwise be tempted to consume.**

Flexible
Fitness Guide

Alcohol Intake

In order to improve your physical wellbeing, you must accept that you need to minimize your consumption of alcohol. It is not good for your organs in the long run and can cause many health complications. An occasional drink is acceptable, but we must stop you if you ever think of going on a college-style binge.

When consuming alcohol, it must fit into your calorie count. To do this, consider the fact that alcohol contains 7 calories per gram. If you are on a gaining regimen, deduct whatever you drink in the form of alcohol from your daily carbohydrate intake. If you are on a fat loss diet with minimal carbohydrates to begin with, deduct the alcohol intake from your daily fat intake.

For example, if you drink 1 shot (1 fl. oz.) of clear vodka, which contains 60 calories, and your daily carbohydrate intake is 200 grams, you would deduct the alcohol calories as follows: 200 grams of carbohydrates is 800 calories, so now you are only allowed to consume 740 calories in carbohydrates. Remember, the alcohol is seriously lacking in nutrients that you may otherwise be consuming with those 60 calories of carbohydrates.

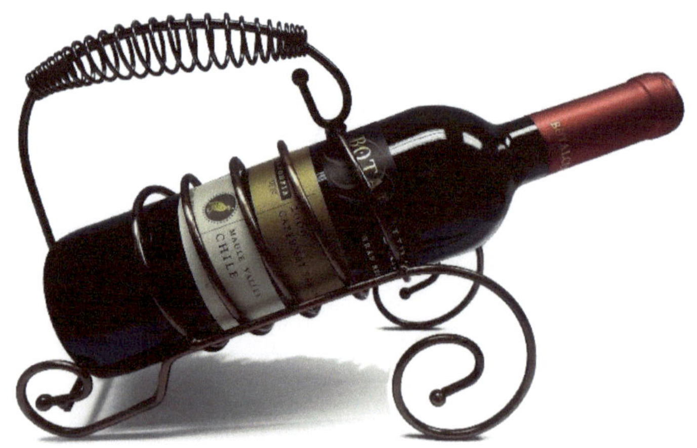

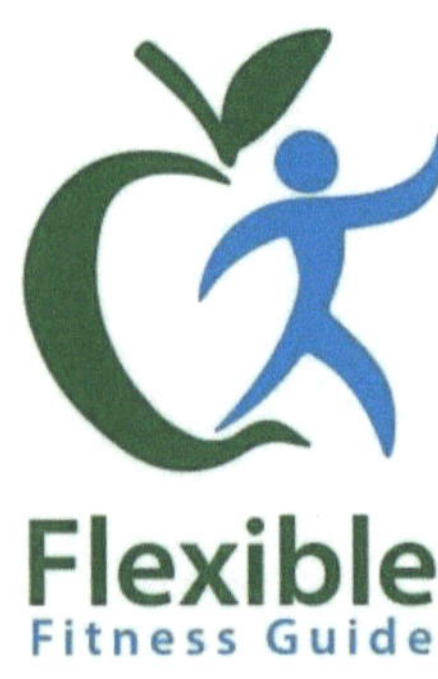

Flexible
Fitness Guide